# KITCHEN MEDS

## EDIBLE AND MEDICINAL PLANTS FOR VIRAL RESPIRATORY INFECTIONS

### Pandemic Edition

## ANNE ANGELONE, MSTCM, DACM, L.AC.

# Table of Contents

# Preface

As COVID-19 becomes endemic, vaccines, face masks, social distancing, and isolation may still go a long way toward managing the virus and its many mutations. However, even if we've applied all these measures, we are still at risk of breakthrough infections. Since vaccines et al measures don't offer complete protection, it seems wise to step up our prevention and treatment strategies. For example, we can learn about and implement the best foods, herbs, and supplements for prevention and the infection's early, middle, and recovery phases.

In my experience of treating thousands of people over several decades, many medicinal herbs can help prevent and mitigate symptoms of viral respiratory infections. In addition, incorporating foods high in flavonoids and other phytonutrients can lend a synergistic effect. To be clear, diet and herbal medicine are not substitutes for vaccines and appropriate medical intervention. Instead, you will discover many medicinal herbs and foods that can be used along with vaccines to help support the immune system. This combined dietary and herbal approach, used for centuries in China, may add an extra layer of protection required to navigate this new frontier of viral respiratory infections.

This guide is for those who want to learn about the most potent medicinal herbs and foods to combat viral respiratory infections. However, it's not for lightweights. The following information is grounded in current research and heavily referenced for you to check out the latest studies. Are you ready to dive in? Excellent. Let's go!

# Phytonutrient Stars

This guide will explore the important role of phytonutrients in managing viral respiratory infections. Phytonutrients are the chemicals produced by plants to protect themselves against the environment. Fortunately, when humans eat fruits and vegetables, these protective benefits are graciously bestowed to the host - that would be you. Importantly, phytonutrients are considered the crown jewels of the plant world since they have well-studied benefits for multiple health conditions, including viral respiratory infections. For example, flavonoids are phytonutrients known for their antioxidant, antimicrobial, anti-inflammatory, and immune-modulating effects that have been extensively investigated for viral respiratory infections (Patel et al., 2018; Eng et al., 2019; Huang et al., 2020; Zakaryan et al., 2017; Ding et al., 2018). Flavonoids are a large family of polyphenolic compounds that make up the plant pigments in fruits, vegetables, and medicinal herbs. Flavonoids are further subdivided according to their structure and include flavonols, flavones, isoflavones, flavanones, flavan3-ols, and anthocyanidins/anthocyanins (aka flavonals).

For clarity's sake, polyphenolic compounds refer to several classes of phytonutrients, including flavonoids, phenolic acids, stilbenes, and lignans. The flavonoids that we will review include flavonols (quercetin,  isorhamnetin, kaempferol, myricetin, rutin) flavones (apigenin, luteolin, baicalin), flavanones (naringenin, hesperetin, hesperidin), isoflavones (daidzein), and flavan-3-ols (catechins and epigallocatechin).

We will also review other phytonutrients such as resveratrol (a stilbene found in red wine and berries), curcumin (a curcuminoid found in turmeric), isoliquiritigenin (a chalcone found in licorice root), and gingerol (a phenolic compound found in ginger). In addition, terpenoids are another important group of phytonutrients for respiratory infections. Terpenoids are a class of hydrocarbons, including terpenes, diterpenes, triterpenes, and sesquiterpenes, with antiviral, antibacterial, antifungal, and immunomodulatory effects (Brahkshatriya et al., 2013).

These phytonutrients, easily sourced from medicinal herbs and everyday foods, have multiple properties, making them stellar candidates for viral respiratory infections. For example, research shows that phytonutrients can modulate multiple cellular pathways, including toll-like receptor (TLR) activation (on innate immune cells) and other signaling pathways responsible for modulating pro-inflammatory cytokines and inflammation (Azam et al., 2019). Phytonutrients can also modulate mast cells, macrophages, lymphocytes, and neutrophil production. In addition, phytonutrients inhibit pro-inflammatory enzymes, including phospholipase A2, cyclooxygenase (COX), lipoxygenase (LOX), and inducible nitric oxide synthase (iNOS). Moreover, phytonutrients upregulate superoxide dismutase and glutathione expression (Gonzalez et al., 2011).

Besides their antioxidant, anti-inflammatory, and immune-modulating effects, many phytonutrients demonstrate antiviral activity against SARS-CoV-2. We know this because of computational chemical biology techniques (such as molecular docking), which have allowed researchers to screen potential natural compounds for managing COVID-19 (Ren et al., 2020). For example, research suggests that common flavonoids, such as kaempferol, luteolin and quercetin, scutellarin and baicalin, naringenin, rutin, apigenin, oleuropein, curcumin, catechin, epigallocatechin gallate (ECGC), gingerol, may all help block viral entry and inhibit viral replication of SARS-CoV-2  (Zhang et al., 2020; Chen & Du, 2020; Niu et al., 2020; Khaerunnisa et al., 2020).

Separately, a computational study by Allam et al., 2020 found that gingerol, curcumin, and allicin interacted with proteins of both SARS-CoV-2 and ACE2 receptors and might have a role in impeding SARS-CoV-2 replication. In addition, one of the most promising terpenoids is glycyrrhizin from licorice root, which is also predicted to bind with the ACE2 receptor to block SARS-CoV-2 entry (Chen & Du, 2020). All of these effects make phytonutrients important players in viral respiratory infections.

As you read through this guide, remember that when we consume phytonutrients, such as flavonoids, phenolic acids, stilbenes, and lignans in fruits, vegetables, and medicinal herbs, they have beneficial antioxidant, anti-inflammatory, immune-modulating, and antiviral effects, required for viral respiratory infections. This exciting information should help you strategize a plant-forward (i.e., phytonutrient-rich) diet for your prevention and treatment strategy. The following chart includes some of the most promising antioxidant, anti-inflammatory, immune-modulating, and antiviral compounds easily sourced from everyday foods.

| Flavonoids, Curcuminoids, and Terpenoids in Everyday Foods | | |
|---|---|---|
| **Flavonoid Category** | **Flavonoid Name** | **Example foods containing these compounds** |
| **Flavonols** | Quercetin | Red and yellow onions, capers, oregano, cloves, elderberry |

| | Kaempferol | Tea, brassicas (broccoli, kale, brussels sprouts, cabbage), chives, spinach, endive, leeks, tomatoes |
|---|---|---|
| | Myricetin | Red wine, grapes, leaves of sweet potato, parsley, tea, blueberries |
| | Rutin | Buckwheat, apples, tea |
| **Flavones** | | |
| | Apigenin | Parsley, celery, olive oil |

| | | |
|---|---|---|
| | Luteolin | Oregano, chamomile, olives, olive oil, artichokes, radicchio, green peppers |
| | Baicalein | Spring onions |
| **Flavanones** | | |
| | Hesperetin<br><br>Hesperidin<br><br>Naringenin | Oranges, grapefruit, lemons, lime |
| **Flavan-3-ols** | | |
| | Catechin<br><br>Epicatechin<br><br>ECGC | Cocoa, prune juice, green tea, white tea, oolong, black tea, grapes, plums, wine, apple juice, lentils, almond, hazelnuts |

| **Anthocyanidins** *(flavonals)* Anthocyanins | Cyanidin Delphinidin Malvidin Pelargonidin Peonidin Petunidin | Cocoa, red wine, grapes, berries, cherries, peach, red apple, pear, peach, plums |
|---|---|---|
| **Isoflavones** | Daidzein Genistein | Soy, alfalfa sprouts, red clover, chickpeas, peanuts, kudzu |
| **Stilbenes** | Resveratrol | Lingonberries, red wine, grapes, peanuts |
| **Lignans** | Lignans | Flax seeds, sesame seeds, soybeans, cruciferous veggies, apricots, strawberries |

| **Curcuminoids** | | |
|---|---|---|
| | Curcumin | Turmeric |
| **Terpenoids** | | |
| | Glycyrrhizin | Licorice root |
| **Polyphenolic Compounds** | | |
| | Gingerol | Ginger |
| | Oleuropein | Olive oil |

| Polyphenols & phenolic acids | | |
|---|---|---|
| | Chrysin<br><br>Caffeic acid<br><br>Galangin<br><br>Hesperidin | Honey |
| | Chlorogenic acid Diterpenes<br>Trigonelline | Coffee |
| **Organosulfur Compounds** | | |
| | Allicin | Garlic |

As we advance, we will review multiple phytonutrients in edible and medicinal plants that demonstrate antioxidant, anti-inflammatory, immune-modulating, and antiviral activity. Remember that phytonutrients are powerful because they act on multiple cellular pathways that regulate the immune system and inflammation, making them ideal candidates for viral respiratory infections and overall health. Let's begin by reviewing the most promising phytonutrients in medicinal herbs and everyday foods that possess antiviral effects.

# Antiviral Compounds in Herbs and Foods

In addition to their antioxidant, anti-inflammatory, and immune-modulating effects, we now know that specific phytonutrients also demonstrate antiviral activity. We know this because researchers and drug companies have screened herbal compounds with antiviral activity for several decades. Plant compounds must interfere with the viral attachment, entry, and replication process to be considered effective antivirals. For example, molecular docking studies predict that the most promising phytonutrients for inhibiting the main protease (Mpro) responsible for viral replication in SARS-CoV-2 include kaempferol, luteolin, quercetin, apigenin, naringenin, oleuropein, curcumin, catechin, epigallocatechin gallate (ECGC), baicalin, baicalein, gingerol, and allicin (Khaerunnisa et al., 2020; Allam et al., 2020; Liu et al., 2021). As the chart above shows, these phytonutrients can easily be sourced from food. For example, from start to finish, capers, oregano, onions, parsley, citrus, olive oil, turmeric, green tea, ginger, and garlic cover this list of phytonutrients.

In another molecular docking study, Tallei et al. (2020) found that hesperidin, cannabinoids, morin, rhoifolin, and ECGC had better binding with the main protease (Mpro) and spike (S) proteins of SARS-CoV-2. Hesperidin is a flavanone found in citrus, mint, and chrysanthemums. Cannabinoids include cannabidiol and tetrahydrocannabinol from Cannabis Sativa and Cannabis Indica. Morin is a flavone found in Folium Mori (Mulberry leaf), almonds, old fustic, and guava. Rhoifolin is a flavone found in bitter oranges, bergamot, grapefruit, lemon, tomatoes, artichokes, bananas, and grapes. Epigallocatechin gallate (ECGC) is a flavon-3-ol found in green tea, apple skins, plums, onions, and hazelnuts.

Other studies show that rutin, a flavonol, is also predicted to inhibit the main protease (Mpro) responsible for SARS-CoV-2 replication (Das et al., 2020). Rutin is found in apples, buckwheat, tea, and medicinal herbs used for respiratory infections, such as Radix Glehniae, Folium Mori, and Fructus Forsythiae. Interestingly, researchers also found that certain flavonoids, such as hesperetin, are predicted to bind with the ACE2 receptor to block SARS-CoV-2 entry (Chen & Du, 2020). Hesperetin is found in dietary and medicinal herbs such as dried citrus peel (Pericarpium Citri Reticulatae), mint (Herba Menthae), and chrysanthemum flower (Flos Chrysanthemi). Researchers also showed that the structure of ACE2 and spike protein fragments becomes unstable in the presence of the flavanone hesperidin (Basu et al., 2020).

Meanwhile, isorhamnetin, a methylated quercetin derivative, demonstrated the most potent binding potential to both ACE2 and the main protease (Mpro) site of SARS-CoV-2. Isorhamnetin is found in sea buckthorn fruit (Hippophae Rhamnoides), yellow onions, parsley, bell peppers, berries, and grapes (Li et al., 2021). Similarly, glyasperin, a methoxyisoflavan found in licorice (Glycyrrhizae Radix et Rhizoma), had the strongest binding activity to ACE site 1 (ibid, 2021).

Separately, gingerol, a phenolic compound in ginger, was shown to bind to and inhibit PLpro, another critical protein involved in SARS-CoV-2 replication (Li et al., 2021).

In addition, Maurya et al. 2020 showed that curcuminoids such as curcumin (found in turmeric) demonstrated strong interaction with the spike (S) protein and ACE2 proteins. Interestingly, SARS-CoV-1 research found that polyphenolic compounds such as Tetra- O-galloyl-β-D-glucose (TGG) from Galla Chinensis and luteolin extracted from medicinal herbs were shown to bind with the surface spike (S2) protein of SARS-CoV-1 to block entry into the host cell (Yi et al., 2004). Given the homology of SARS-CoV-1 and SARS-CoV-2, researchers suspect that herbs containing these compounds are potential candidates that may help inhibit the main protease (Mpro) and spike protein in SARS-CoV-2.

Separately, daidzein was also shown to inhibit the main protease (Mpro) of SARS-CoV-1 (Nguyen et al., 2012; Schwarz et al., 2014). Daidzein is an isoflavone abundant in soy, especially tempeh. Other foods that contain smaller amounts of daidzein include common black beans and peanuts.

Finally, geniposide in Gardenia Jasminoides targets another SARS-CoV-2 protease, TMPRSS2, which may also help inhibit viral entry into host cells (Li et al., 2021). This research suggests the antiviral potential of each of these phytochemicals to interfere with SARS-CoV-2. This information should help you recognize the flavonoids and specific foods to include in your diet.

In addition to those already presented, the following chart summarizes compounds in herbs and foods that may interfere with viral attachment, entry, and replication. As you read through each section, consider the phytonutrients with antiviral effects on multiple pathways. For example, epigallocatechin gallate (ECGC) in green tea might help inhibit the main protease (Mpro) and spike (S) proteins of SARS-CoV-2.

| Phytonutrients That Might Help Inhibit SARS-CoV-2 | | |
| --- | --- | --- |
| ACE2 blockade | Phytonutrients | Examples of dietary and medicinal plants that contain these compounds. |
| | Glycyrrhizin/Glyasperin | Licorice |
| | Hesperetin | Pericarpium Citri Reticulatae |
| | Chlorogenic Acid | Honeysuckle |
| | Forsythoside A | Fructus Forsythiae |
| | Patchouli alcohol | Herba Pogostemonis |
| | Emodin | |

| | Isorhamnetin | Rhubarb root |
|---|---|---|
| | Resveratrol | Sea buckthorn fruit |
| | Scutellarin | Polygonum Cuspidatum |
| | Hesperedin | Skullcap |
| | Gingerol | Fructus Aurantii Immaturus |
| | Curcumin | Ginger |
| | Allicin | Turmeric |
| | | Garlic |
| M^pro inhibition | Quercetin, quercetrin, and cinanserin | Houttuynia Cordata |
| | Kaempferol | Dryopteris Crassirhizoma |
| | Baicalein | Skullcap |
| | Hesperidin and neohesperidin | Fructus Aurantii Immaturus |
| | ECGC | Green tea |
| | Allicin | Garlic |
| | Curcumin | Turmeric |
| | Gingerol | Ginger |
| | Apigenin | Chrysanthemum |
| | Luteolin | Honeysuckle |
| | Naringenin | Pericarpium Citri Reticulatae |
| | Myristicin | Nutmeg |
| | Eugenol | Clove |
| | Morin | Mulberry leaf |
| | Rhoifolin | Bitter orange |
| | Patchouli alcohol | Herba Pogostemonis |
| | Rutin | Fructus Forsythiae |
| | Sinigrin, β-sitosterol, and indigo | Isatis Indigotica |
| | Cannabinoids | Cannabis spp. |
| | 2β-hydroxy-3,4-seco-friedelolactone- | Herba Violae |

| | 27-oic acid, isodecortinol, and cerevisterol | |
| --- | --- | --- |
| **PL$^{pro}$ inhibition** | Platycodin D | Radix Platycodi |
| | Baicalin | Skullcap |
| | Gingerol | Ginger root |
| | Phaitanthrin D and 2,2-di (3-indolyl)-3-indolone | Isatis Indigotica |
| **Spike protein binding** | Quercetin | Houttuynia Cordata |
| | Luteolin | Herba Violae |
| | Tetra-O-galloyl-β-D-glucose (TGG) | Galla Chinensis |
| | Chlorogenic Acid | Honeysuckle |
| | Morin | Mulberry leaf |
| | ECGC | Green tea |
| | Myristicin | Nutmeg |
| | Eugenol | Clove |
| | Rhoifolin | Bitter orange |
| | Hesperidin | Fructus Aurantii Immaturus |
| | Cannabinoids | Cannabis spp. |
| | Curcumin | Turmeric |

| | | |
|---|---|---|
| **Helicase inhibition** | Scutellarein<br><br>Hesperidin | Skullcap<br><br>Fructus Aurantii Immaturus |
| **RNA- dependent RNA polymerase (RdRp) inhibition** | Quercetin<br><br>Quercetrin,<br><br>Cinanserin | Houttuynia Cordata |
| **Viroporin 3a ion channel inhibition** | Emodin | Rhubarb root |
| **TMPRSS2 inhibition** | Geniposide<br><br>Platycodon D<br><br>Andrographolide | Gardenia Jasminoides<br><br>Radix Platycodi<br><br>Andrographis Paniculata* |

Sources (Khaerunnisa et al., 2020; Li et al., 2021; Tallei et al., 2020; Wu et al., 2020; Das et al., 2020). *Avoid the use of this herb in autoimmune conditions.

Now that you know more about the antiviral effects of specific herbs and everyday foods let's continue to explore the anti-inflammatory and immune-modulating effects of phytonutrients.

# Anti-Inflammatory and Immune-Modulating Effects

In addition to their antiviral effects, many phytonutrients also act on a critical gene transcription factor called Nuclear Factor Kappa B (NFKB). NFKB is a protein that turns inflammation either "on" or "off" when cells sense danger in the form of infections. However, if NFKB is overactive, as in the case of respiratory infections, it will continually produce an inflammation response where none is needed. For example, activation of NFKB leads to gene transcription of pro-inflammatory cytokines associated with acute respiratory distress syndrome (ARDS) (Horowitz et al., 2020). In addition, activation of (NLRP3) inflammasome contributes to cytokine production in respiratory distress syndrome associated with SARS coronaviruses (Chen et al., 2019).

In COVID-19 patients, activation of NFKB and the NLRP3 inflammasome can lead to a runaway production of pro-inflammatory cytokines, such as IL-6, TNF-$\alpha$, and IL-1$\beta$, known as the cytokine storm. Since immune activity and inflammation can become excessive in COVID-19 and other viral respiratory infections, including natural agents that modulate NFKB and cytokine overexpression makes sense. Besides appropriate medical intervention, knowing how to counteract this immune-inflammatory cascade with herbs and foods can help all stages of the infection. The critical point is to become aware of and apply the most advanced strategies to effectively tame hyperimmune responses and resultant inflammation.

Fortunately, we now know that phytonutrients in edible and medicinal plants have the power to bind to and "turn off" gene transcription factors like NFKB (which turns off pro-inflammatory cytokines). In addition to the most ubiquitous compounds listed above, several other promising anti-inflammatory phytonutrients act on NFKB. For example, isorhamnetin in sea buckthorn fruit demonstrates antioxidant activities and inhibits the lipopolysaccharide (LPS)-induced inflammatory response via inhibition of NFKB signaling (Shi et al., 2018). Isorhamnetin can also be found in yellow onions, parsley, bell peppers, berries, and grapes.

Separately, baicalein is a flavone in herbs used for respiratory infections, such as Rhizoma Pinelliae Preparata and Scutellaria Baicalensis. Baicalein has well-known anti-inflammatory and immune-modulating effects and has been shown to inhibit the activation of NFKB and decrease TNF-$\alpha$ and IL-6 (Xu et al., 2019). Baicalein is also abundant in spring onions (Cheng et al., 2018).

Acetoside, a phenylethanoid glycoside, relieved LPS-induced acute lung injury by inhibiting pro-inflammatory cytokines and NFKB activation in vitro and in vivo studies (Jing et al., 2015). Acetoside can be found in Verbena, Lemon Verbena, and olives. Similarly, nobiletin, a flavone in citrus peel (Pericarpium Citri Reticulatae), ameliorates inflammation in acute lung injury by suppressing the NFKB pathway in vivo and in vitro (Li et al., 2018).

In addition, gingerol, a phenolic compound in ginger, has anti-inflammatory and immune-modulating effects, such as reducing the synthesis of pro-inflammatory cytokines TNF-$\alpha$, IL-1, and IL-8, via suppressing NFKB activation (Mashhadi et al., 2013). Shogaol, another phenolic compound in ginger, also has potent anti-inflammatory effects, while allicin inhibits influenza A (H1N1) neuraminidase, demonstrating its antiviral effects (Sahoo et al., 2016).

Finally, you'll remember that resveratrol is an NFKB-inhibiting polyphenol abundant in grapes, red wine, peanuts, and Itadori tea (Polygonum Cuspidatum). The most promising phytonutrients that may help inhibit NFKB, cytokines, and inflammation induced by SARS-CoV-2 include kaempferol, luteolin, quercetin, acetoside, isorhamnetin, nobiletin, baicalein, gingerol, and resveratrol, which can also be sourced from dietary herbs and foods (Li et al., 2018; Li et al., 2021). Multiple flavonoids such as wogonoside, baicalin, kaempferol, luteolin, myricetin, quercetin, and apigenin have also been shown to interfere with NLRP3 inflammasome signaling, thereby alleviating the inflammatory response to SARS-CoV-2 infection (McKee et al., 2020). Given these beneficial effects, we can consider sourcing phytonutrients from food and herbal medicine that "turn off" NFKB and interfere with NLRP3 inflammasome signaling. In addition to those already considered, the following chart includes examples of herbs and foods that you can include in your prevention and treatment plan.

| Natural NFKB Inhibitors | |
|---|---|
| • Allicin in garlic | • Sulforaphane in cruciferous vegetables |
| • Curcumin in turmeric | • Vitamins A, C, D, E |
| • Epigallocatechin gallate (ECGC) and theanine in green tea | • Berberine in Coptis Rhizoma |
| • Ginkgolides in gingko biloba | • Kaempferol in spinach, kale, chives |
| • Melatonin in mushrooms | • Luteolin in celery, broccoli, cabbage |
| • Lipoic acid in spinach, broccoli, yams | • Quercetin in leeks, citrus, spinach |
| • Acetoside in Lemon Verbena, olive | • Zinc in oysters, crab, shrimp |
| • Silymarin in milk thistle | • EPA/DHA in fish and algae |
| • Carnosol in rosemary | • Gingerols in ginger |
| • Selenium in cod, shrimp, salmon, tuna, button mushrooms | • Baicalin in Scutellaria Baicalensis |
| • Limonene in lemongrass, lemon, orange, and grapefruit essential oils | • Alpha-pinene in pine, sage, and eucalyptus essential oils |
| • Resveratrol in grapes, red wine, peanuts, Itadori tea | • Isorhametin in sea buckthorn, yellow onions, parsley, bell peppers, berries, grapes |

| Natural NLRP3 Inhibitors | |
| --- | --- |
| • Wogonoside and baicalin in Scutellaria Baicalensis | • Quercetin in black elderberry, oregano, capers |
| • Apigenin in parsley, celery, olive oil | • Kaempferol in spinach, kale, chives |
| • Myricetin in red wine, grapes, blueberries, parsley, green and black tea | • Luteolin in celery, broccoli, cabbage |

These potent compounds help inhibit NFKB and NLRP3, which can result in less inflammation and overall symptom improvement. Besides respiratory illnesses all of these natural inhibitors may be helpful for all inflammatory conditions.


## The Takeaway

We have established that multiple foods and traditional herbs provide a rich source of therapeutic agents for viral respiratory infections. Many of these foods and herbs contain compounds with antioxidant, antiviral, anti-inflammatory, and immune-modulating activity. Considering these effects, you can imagine how combining phytonutrients from foods and medicinal herbs can help combat viral respiratory infections. The more we understand each plant's constituents and actions, the more we can strategize the synergistic use of herbs and foods to support our immune system and improve our health.

# The Gut-Lung Axis

Intriguingly, research has shed light on the crosstalk between gut microbiota and the lungs, known as the gut–lung axis. For example, extensive studies have observed alterations in gut microbial species (and their toxic metabolites) in lung diseases, including pneumonia, asthma, allergy, and lung cancer (Zhang et al., 2020). Microbial dysbiosis in the gut combined with a pro-inflammatory diet can break down the integrity of the mucosal barrier and lead to the translocation of bacteria and their metabolites into the systemic circulation, setting the stage for adaptive immune cell activation and more inflammation. However, we also know that flavonoid consumption regulates gut bacteria by stimulating the growth of good flora and inhibiting harmful bacteria, which modulate intestinal and systemic inflammation and the metabolic response (Cassidy & Minehane, 2017). Herbal medicine also promotes the growth of good flora by acting as prebiotics (Singdevsachan et al., 2016).

Since alterations in gut bacteria have subsequently been linked to immune-inflammation responses and lung disease development, consuming more flavonoids may be a viable strategy to manipulate the gut microbiota as a therapeutic approach for lung diseases (Zhang et al., 2020). Importantly, multiple flavonoids can all be sourced from our diets and herbal medicine to promote the production of good flora. After absorption, these phytochemicals also help improve gut barrier integrity by inducing the expressions of tight junction proteins (Carrasco-Pozo, 2013). In addition, all of these compounds demonstrate antiviral activity and regulate a wide range of signaling pathways, such as NFKB and cytokines, which leads to their anti-inflammatory and immune-modulating effects.

# Functional Flavonoids

Foods that create a beneficial physiologic response in the body are called functional foods. The most potent flavonoids that demonstrate antiviral, anti-inflammatory, and immune-modulating effects include quercetin, kaempferol, rutin, luteolin, apigenin, hesperetin, hesperidin, and baicalin. Considering this activity, consuming edible and medicinal plants rich in these and other potent phytonutrients may provide a novel strategy for preventing and managing viral respiratory diseases, including COVID-19.

In studying the foods that contain these compounds, astute patients can consider using foods like practitioners recommend herbal medicines. For example, we can understand what's required to decrease inflammation and balance the immune system, then find the plants containing the specific compounds to accomplish this task. Let's now explore the most potent and ubiquitous phytonutrients in our diets and their benefits, keeping in mind that they all regulate multiple pathways involved in viral respiratory diseases.

## Quercetin

Quercetin is one of the most ubiquitous antiviral, anti-inflammatory, and immune-modulating flavonols found in everyday food such as apples, grapes, onions, citrus, and dietary herbs used for viral respiratory infections such as red dates, chrysanthemum, and honeysuckle. Consuming more quercetin-rich foods may be as important as herbal remedies for their antiviral, anti-inflammatory, and immune-modulating effects. For example, quercetin affects immunity and inflammation by acting mainly on leukocytes and targeting intracellular signaling kinases, enzymes, and membrane proteins crucial for cellular-specific functions (Chirimbolo, 2010).

Quercetin also has a protective effect on cells and has been shown to successfully attenuate oxidative epithelial cell injury in lung inflammation (Hayashi et al., 2012). In addition, quercetin can suppress NLRP3 inflammasome activation (Choe & Kim, 2017). You will recall that Khaerunnisa et al. (2020) found that quercetin was predicted to inhibit the main protease (Mpro) responsible for viral replication in SARS-CoV-2. In addition, quercetin has also been shown to interfere with spike protein binding, ACE2, and other viral proteins such as RdRp and PLpro, indicating its massive antiviral potential against SARS-CoV-2 (Huang et al., 2020).

While we can't be certain that quercetin will block entry and inhibit viral replication of SARS-CoV-2 as predicted, we know that combining flavonoid-rich foods and herbs is undoubtedly beneficial for the gut microbiome and lung health.

The following chart highlights commonly used herbs that contain quercetin. All herbs in this chart are routinely recommended by Traditional Chinese Medicine (TCM) herbalists for viral respiratory infections. While these herbs are generally recognized as safe, it's essential to consult with an herbalist when using herbs in combination.

## Herbs That Contain Quercetin

| | |
|---|---|
| • Herba Ephedrae | • Eriobotryae Folium |
| • Toona Sinensis Roem | • Zizyphus Jujubae |
| • Herba Violae | • Houttuynia Cordata |
| • Herba Menthae | • Flos Chrysanthemi |
| • Rhizoma Polygonum Cuspidatum | • Folium Mori |
| • Flos Lonicerae Japonicae | • Radix et Rhizoma Asteris |
| • Fructus Forsythiae | • Rhodiola Crenulata |

## Foods That Contain Quercetin

The following chart highlights many common foods that contain quercetin, which you are encouraged to include more of in your diet for their antiviral, anti-inflammatory, and immune-modulating effects for respiratory infections. Notably, the first thirty-nine foods on this list are among the top 100 nutrient-dense foods featured in the Guide to Nutrivore (Ballantyne, 2022). Making the top 100 list reflects the fact that these foods are nutritional powerhouses with multiple health benefits beyond their flavonoid content.

## Quercetin-Rich Foods

| | |
|---|---|
| • Watercress | • Strawberries |
| • Mustard greens | • Tomatoes* |
| • Collards | • Green beans |
| • Parsley | • Fennel |
| • Bok Choy | • Butternut squash |
| • Kale | • Sweet potatoes |
| • Arugula | • Oranges |
| • Spinach | • Black elderberry |
| • Broccoli | • Oregano |

| | |
|---|---|
| • Black tea | • Mint |
| • Basil | • Capers |
| • Green tea | • Cloves |
| • Brussels sprouts | • Shallots |
| • Cilantro | • Red onion |
| • Red Leaf lettuce | • Bilberry |
| • Green Leaf lettuce | • Red wine |
| • Butterhead lettuce | • Grapefruit |
| • Radicchio | • Cranberries |
| • Turnip | • Apples |
| • Rhubarb | • Yellow onions |
| • Spring onions | • Pomegranate |
| • Cocoa, unsweetened | • Sorrel |
| • Asparagus | • Dill |
| • Asian pears | • Okra |
| • Summer squash | • Leeks |
| • Mung bean sprouts | • Ginger |
| • Alfalfa sprouts | • Sage |
| • Zucchini squash | • Fennel leaves |
| • Iceberg lettuce | • Cherries |
| • Lychee fruit | • Blueberries |
| • Tomatillos* | • Mulberries |
| • Blackberries | • Figs |
| | • Grapes |
| | • Guava |
| | • Papaya |
| | • Mango |

Sources: (Ballantyne, 2022; Miean & Mohammad, 2001; Bhagwat et al., 2011; Dabeek & Marra 2019; USDA (US Department of Agriculture) Database for the Flavonoid Content of Selected Foods; Phenol Explorer).

Here is a visual guide of quercetin-rich foods to include in your diet. From top to bottom, this includes watercress, mustard greens, collards, Bok choy, kale, arugula, spinach, broccoli, basil, Brussels sprouts, cilantro, red leaf lettuce, green leaf lettuce, radicchio, turnip, and rhubarb.

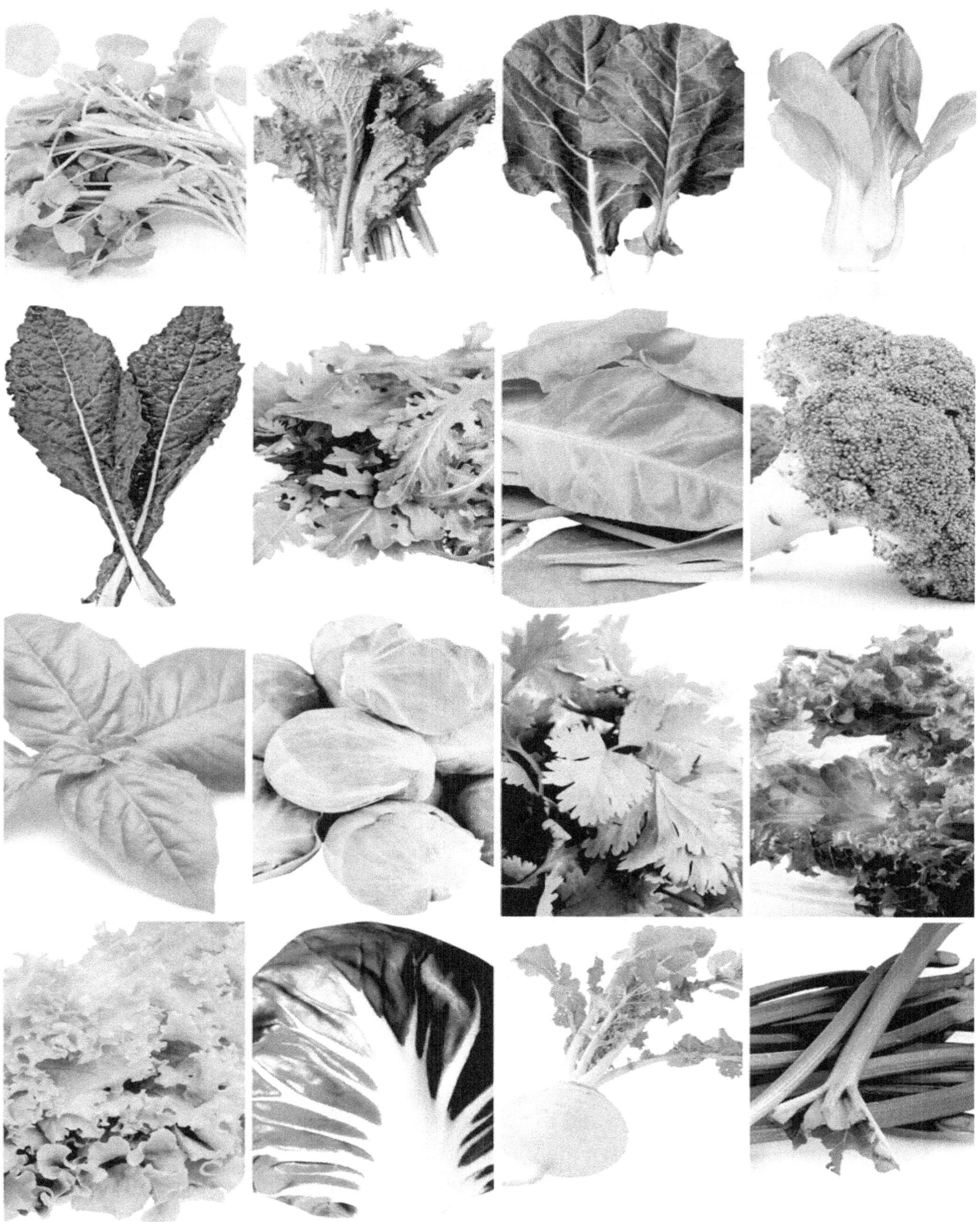

## Kaempferol

Kaempferol is a flavonol found in many common foods, such as capers, cabbage, spinach, and broccoli. Kaempferol is also abundant in medicinal herbs historically used for viral respiratory infections, such as Folium Mori (Mulberry leaf), Fructus Forsythiae (Forsythia), and Herba Menthae (Mint). Consuming more kaempferol-rich foods may be as important as herbal remedies for their antiviral, anti-inflammatory, and immune-modulating effects. For example, kaempferol exhibits anti-inflammatory actions by inhibiting phospholipase A2 (via arachidonic acid), lipoxygenase (LOX), cyclooxygenase (COX), thromboxane enzymes, and the inhibition of inducible nitric oxide synthase (iNOS) and nitric oxide (NO) (Santangelo et al., 2007; Yoon & Baek, 2005). Significantly, kaempferol can attenuate LPS-induced acute lung injury via inhibiting MAPK and NFKB signaling pathways (Chen et al., 2012). Kaempferol also acts on TNF-α to modulate systemic inflammation and oxidative stress (Yang et al., 2015).

In addition to kaempferol's anti-inflammatory and immune-modulating effects, it also demonstrates antiviral activity, making it another stellar candidate for viral respiratory infections. For example, a molecular docking study by Khaerunnisa et al. (2020) found that kaempferol could inhibit the main protease (Mpro) responsible for viral replication in SARS-CoV-2. While we can't be sure that kaempferol from herbs and foods will block the main protease (Mpro) of SARS-CoV-2 as predicted, we know that consuming phytonutrient-rich foods and herbs is beneficial for the gut microbiome and lung health.

The following chart highlights many herbs that contain kaempferol. TCM herbalists commonly recommend all of these herbs for viral respiratory infections. While these herbs are generally recognized as safe, it's important to consult with a trained herbalist when using herbs in combination for each stage of infection.

| Herbs That Contain Kaempferol | |
| --- | --- |
| • Folium Mori | • Fructus Forsythiae |
| • Dryopteris Crassirhizoma | • Flos Lonicerae Japonicae |
| • Herba Ephedrae | • Flos Chrysanthemi |
| • Herba Menthae | • Rhodiola Crenulata |
| • Eriobotryae Folium | • Armeniacae Amarum |

## Foods That Contain Kaempferol

As part of your prevention strategy and to potentiate the effect of herbal remedies, you can also focus on consuming foods rich in kaempferol. Importantly, the first forty-two foods on this list are among most nutrient-dense foods featured in the Guide to Nutrivore (Ballantyne, 2022).

# Kaempferol-Rich Foods

- Mustard greens
- Collards
- Swiss Chard
- Bok Choy
- Kale
- Arugula
- Spinach
- Broccoli
- Black Tea
- Radish
- Basil
- Green Tea
- Brussels sprouts
- Endive
- Red Leaf Lettuce
- Green Cabbage
- Red Cabbage
- Kohlrabi
- Rutabaga
- Chives
- Green Leaf Lettuce
- Butterhead Lettuce

- Blackberries
- Strawberries
- Tomatillos*
- Green beans
- Carrots
- Butternut squash
- Sweet potatoes
- Kiwi, golden
- Capers
- Dill
- Napa cabbage
- Turnip greens
- Leeks
- Radish sprouts
- Tarragon
- Saffron
- Mint
- Cumin
- Cloves
- Caraway
- Ginger
- Green onions

- Peas, podded
- Red Bell Pepper*
- Asparagus
- Spring Onions
- Asian Pears
- Summer Squash
- Mung bean sprouts
- Alfalfa sprouts
- Zucchini squash
- Celery
- Iceberg Lettuce
- Tomatoes*

- Sorrel
- Chicory
- Leeks
- Savoy Cabbage
- Onions
- Lotus root
- Potatoes*
- Almonds
- Apples
- Red raspberry
- Blueberries
- Gooseberries
- Elderberries
- Watermelon
- Peaches
- Apricots
- Cherries
- Red wine

Sources: (Ballantyne, 2022; Phenol Explorer; Miean & Mohammad, 2001; Bhagwat et al., 2011; Dabeek & Marra 2019; USDA (US Department of Agriculture) Database for the Flavonoid Content of Selected Foods). *Peppers, tomatoes, tomatillos, and potatoes contain the glycoalkaloid solanine, which may cause inflammation in some individuals. Below is a visual guide of kaempferol-rich foods to include in your diet. From top to bottom, this includes watercress, mustard greens, collards, Swiss chard, Bok choy, arugula, spinach, broccoli, black tea, radish, basil, green tea, Brussels sprouts, endive, red leaf lettuce, and green cabbage.

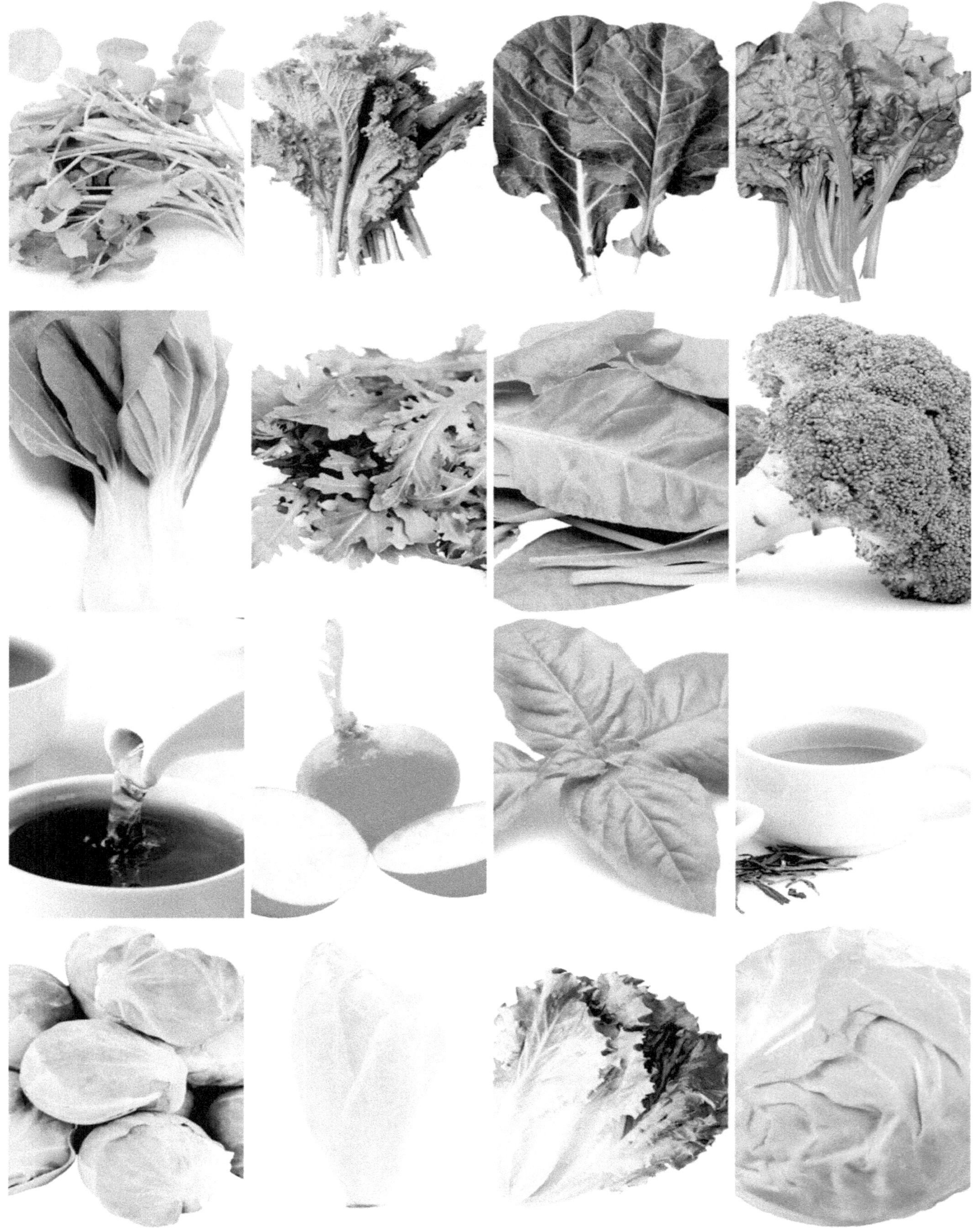

# Rutin

Rutin is a flavonol in many fruits, vegetables, and medicinal herbs such as apples, grapes, capers, buckwheat, and tomatoes. Consuming more rutin-rich foods may also be as important as the herbal remedies for their antiviral, anti-inflammatory, and immune-modulating effects. For example, rutin can inhibit NFKB and modulate the expression of COX-2 in LPS-induced lung injury (Yeh et al., 2014). Rutin also exerts an anti-inflammatory protective effect by decreasing nitric oxide and inhibiting the protein expression levels of TLR4, thereby alleviating lung tissue injury (Tian et al., 2022). In addition to its antioxidant and anti-inflammatory effects, rutin is predicted to inhibit the main protease (Mpro) responsible for SARS-CoV-2 replication (Das et al., 2020).

The following chart highlights many herbs that contain rutin. Herbalists commonly recommend all herbs in this chart for viral respiratory infections. Even though these herbs are generally recognized as safe, it's important to consult with an herbalist when combining herbs, as individual needs are always considered.

| Herbs that Contain Rutin | |
| --- | --- |
| <ul><li>Ledebouriella Divaricata</li><li>Astragalus Membranaceus</li><li>Fructus Forsythiae</li></ul> | <ul><li>Fructus Aurantii Immaturus</li><li>Folium Mori</li><li>Radix Glehniae</li></ul> |

## Foods That Contain Rutin

As part of your prevention and treatment strategy, you can focus on consuming the following foods rich in rutin. Notably, the first eight foods on this list are some of the most nutrient-dense foods featured in the Guide to Nutrivore (Ballantyne, 2022).

| Rutin-Rich Foods | |
| --- | --- |
| Black tea | Grapes |
| Green tea | Green currants |
| Cocoa, unsweetened | Black currants |
| Asparagus | Red currants |
| Mung bean sprouts | Blackberries |
| Zucchini | Buckwheat |

| |
|---|
| <table><tr><td><ul><li>Tomatoes*</li><li>Tomatillos*</li><li>Apples</li><li>Black raspberry</li><li>Red raspberry</li><li>Plums</li><li>Apricots</li></ul></td><td><ul><li>Prunes</li><li>Raisins</li><li>Capers</li><li>Black olives</li><li>Fenugreek</li><li>Marjoram</li></ul></td></tr></table> |
| Sources: (Ballantyne, 2022; Phenol Explorer). *Tomatoes and tomatillos contain the glycoalkaloid solanine which may exacerbate inflammation in some individuals. Below is a visual guide to the top foods on this list that contain rutin. |

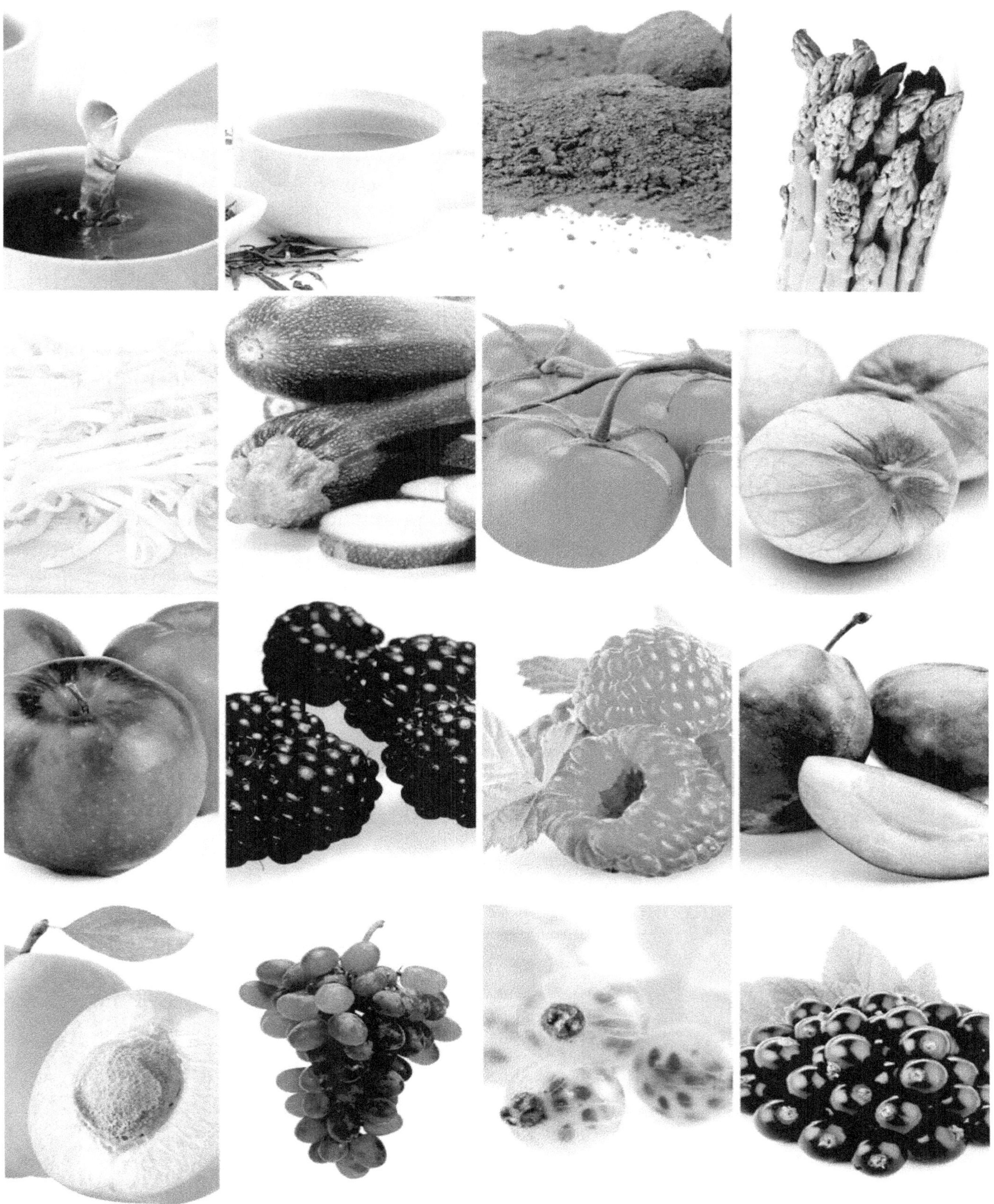

## Luteolin

Luteolin is a flavone in many foods, such as radicchio, chicory, and celery. Luteolin is also abundant in multiple herbs, including Rhodiola species (Zuo et al., 2007), Flos Lonicerae Japonicae (Honeysuckle) (Avendano et al., 2015), Flos Chrysanthemi (Chrysanthemum) (Du et al., 2015), Herba Violae (Peng et al., 2017), Herba Ephedrae (Huang et al., 2020), and Herba Moslae (Hu et al., 2010), among others. Since luteolin has antiviral, immune-modulating, and anti-inflammatory effects, it is an outstanding candidate for viral respiratory infections. For example, luteolin can regulate the pulmonary inflammatory response by suppressing MAPK and NFKB production of TNF-$\alpha$ and IL-6 in endotoxin-induced acute lung injury (Kuo et al., 2011; Kang et al., 2010). In addition, luteolin (and quercetin) can modulate lymphocytes and neutrophils and decrease pro-inflammatory cytokines such as TNF-$\alpha$ and IL-1$\beta$ (Kim et al., 2014). Moreover, luteolin inhibits iNOS and nitric oxide (NO) induced by cytokines (Santangelo et al., 2007). Besides luteolin's anti-inflammatory and immune-modulating effects, luteolin may potentially inhibit the main protease (Mpro) responsible for the viral replication of SARS-CoV-2 (Khaerunnisa et al., 2020).

Considering the heightened immune-inflammatory response in viral respiratory infections and that luteolin suppresses multiple pathways, including NFKB production of pro-inflammatory cytokines, we might consider consuming more luteolin via our diets and herbal medicine to modulate this response. Without further studies, we can't be sure that luteolin from foods and herbs will block entry of the spike protein or inhibit Mpro in SARS-CoV-2 as predicted. However, foods and herbs that contain luteolin are undoubtedly beneficial for the gut microbiome and lung health. The following herbs and foods that contain luteolin can be considered for their antiviral, anti-inflammatory, and immune-modulating effects on viral respiratory illnesses.

All of the herbs in this chart are commonly recommended by herbalists for viral respiratory infections. While these herbs are generally considered safe, remember that it's essential to consult with an herbalist when combining herbs, as individual needs are always considered.

## Herbs That Contain Luteolin

| | |
|---|---|
| • Flos Chrysanthemi | • Rhodiola Crenulata |
| • Herba Moslae | • Flos Lonicerae Japonicae |
| • Herba Ephedrae | • Fructus Forsythiae |
| • Herba Violae | • Houttuynia Cordata |

## Foods That Contain Luteolin

As part of your prevention strategy, and to potentiate the effect of herbal remedies, you can also consume foods rich in luteolin for their antiviral, antioxidant, anti-inflammatory, and immune-modulating effects. Notably, the first twenty-nine foods on this list are among the top 100 nutrient-dense foods featured in the Guide to Nutrivore (Ballantyne, 2022).

<table>
<tr><td colspan="2">

### Luteolin-Rich Foods
</td></tr>
<tr><td>

- Collards
- Swiss Chard
- Parsley
- Spinach
- Broccoli
- Basil
- Brussels sprouts
- Red leaf lettuce
- Green cabbage
- Cauliflower
- Kohlrabi
- Chives
- Green leaf lettuce
- Butterhead lettuce
- Romaine lettuce
- Radicchio
- Spring onions
</td><td>

- Lentils
- Oregano
- Dandelion
- Thyme
- Sage
- Rosemary
- Lemon verbena
- Olives, black
- Olives, green
- Extra virgin olive oil
- Pistachios
- Serrano peppers*
- Chili peppers*
- Chicory greens
- Lemon
- Pumpkin
- Perilla
</td></tr>
</table>

<table>
<tr><td>

- Sweet green peppers*
- Artichokes
- Mung bean sprouts
- Alfalfa sprouts
- Celery
- Iceberg lettuce
- Carrots
- Butternut squash
- Sweet potatoes
- Kiwi, golden
- Oranges

</td><td>

- Cantaloupe
- Watermelon
- Clementines
- Pink and red grapefruit
- Beets
- Blueberries
- Chamomile
- Chrysanthemum
- Dandelion
- Lemongrass
- Leeks
- Tarragon

</td></tr>
</table>

Sources: (Ballantyne, 2022; Dabeek & Marra 2019; Bhagwat et al., 2011; Miean & Mohammad, 2001; Phenol Explorer). *Peppers contain the glycoalkaloid solanine which may cause inflammation in some individuals. Do not use hot peppers should when you have a sore throat.

Below is a visual guide of the top foods on this list that contain luteolin. Here is a visual guide of luteolin-rich foods to include in your diet. From top to bottom, this includes collards, Swiss chard, parsley, spinach, broccoli, basil, Brussels sprouts, red leaf lettuce, green cabbage, cauliflower, rutabaga, chives, green leaf lettuce, butter leaf lettuce, romaine, and radicchio.

 

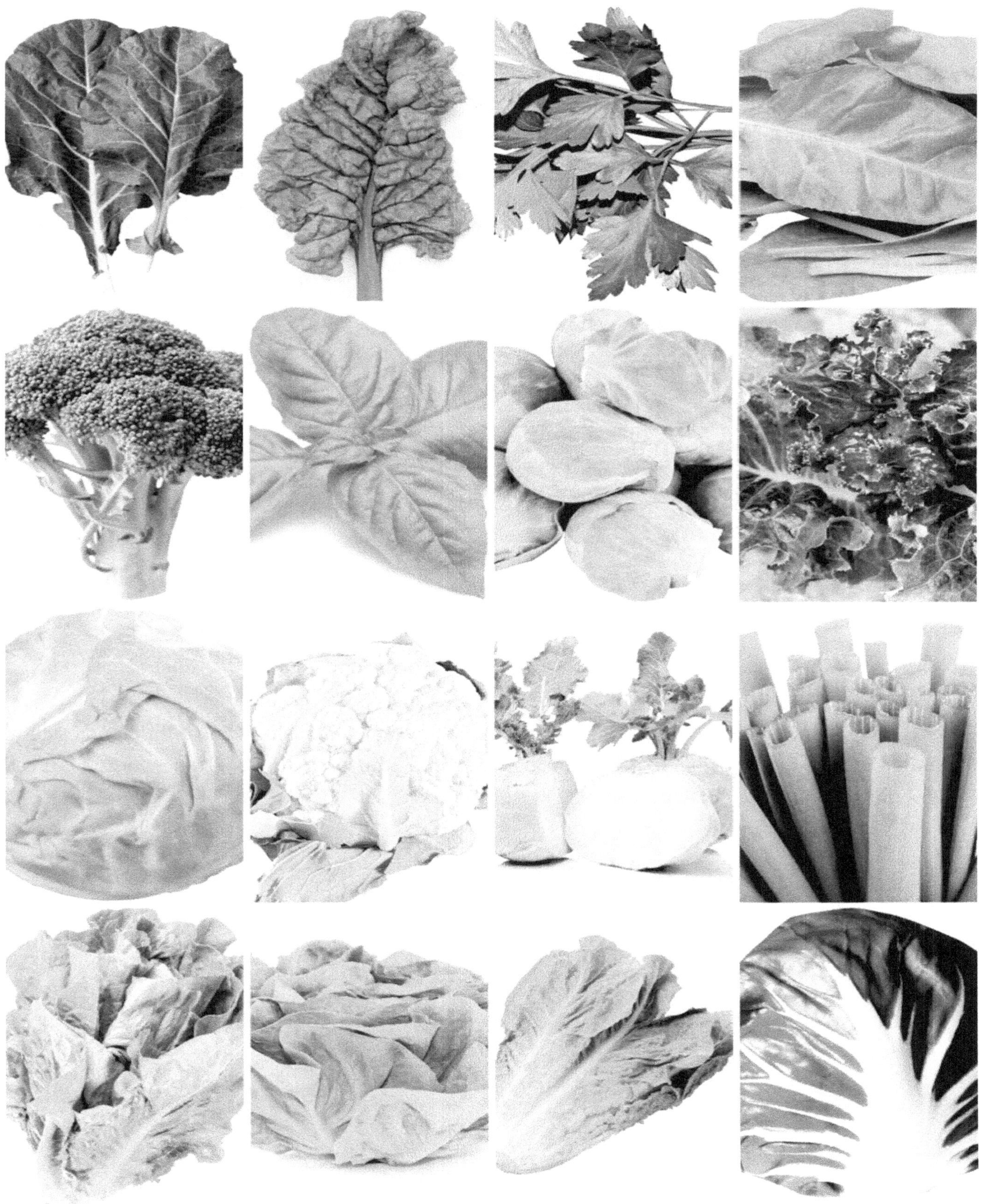

## Apigenin

Apigenin is a flavone found in plants such as parsley, spinach, oregano, peppermint, and chrysanthemum. As with other phytonutrients for viral respiratory infections, consuming more apigenin-rich foods for their antiviral, anti-inflammatory, and immune-modulating effects may be as important as ingesting herbal remedies. For example, you will recall that apigenin demonstrates potential as a main protease (Mpro) inhibitor (Khaerunnisa et al., 2020). Apigenin from chamomile was found to inhibit COX-2 and nitric oxide synthase via inhibition of NFKB (Liang et al., 1999). Apigenin combined with luteolin inhibits human T-cell responses, especially auto-reactive T cells (Verbeek et al., 2004). In addition, apigenin also inhibits the mast cell secretion of histamine, which is generally increased with viral infections (Chirumbulo et al., 2010). All of these effects make apigenin an outstanding candidate for viral respiration infections.

| Herbs that Contain Apigenin | |
| --- | --- |
| • Flos Chrysanthemi<br>• Astragalus Membranaceus | • Herba Menthae<br>• Zizyphus Jujubae |

## Foods That Contain Apigenin

As part of your prevention and treatment strategy, you can also focus on consuming foods rich in apigenin. Notably, the first nine foods on this list are among the most nutrient-dense foods featured in the Guide to Nutrivore (Ballantyne, 2022).

| Apigenin-Rich Foods | |
| --- | --- |
| • Parsley | • Marjoram |
| • Spinach | • Sage |
| • Basil | • Olive oil |
| • Cilantro | • Pistachios |
| • Rutabagas | • Mint |

| | |
|---|---|
| • Spring onions | • Chamomile |
| • Artichokes | • Chrysanthemum |
| • Celery | • Celery seeds |
| • Oranges | • Celery hearts |
| • Tarragon | • Kumquats |
| • Rosemary | • Onions |

Sources: (Ballantyne, 2022; Phenol Explorer; Miean & Mohammad, 2001; Bhagwat et al., 2011; Dabeek & Marra 2019).

Below is a visual guide of apigenin-rich foods to include in your diet. From top to bottom, this includes parsley, spinach, basil, cilantro, rutabaga, spring onions, artichokes, celery, oranges, tarragon, rosemary, oregano, sage, olive oil, pistachios, and mint.

     

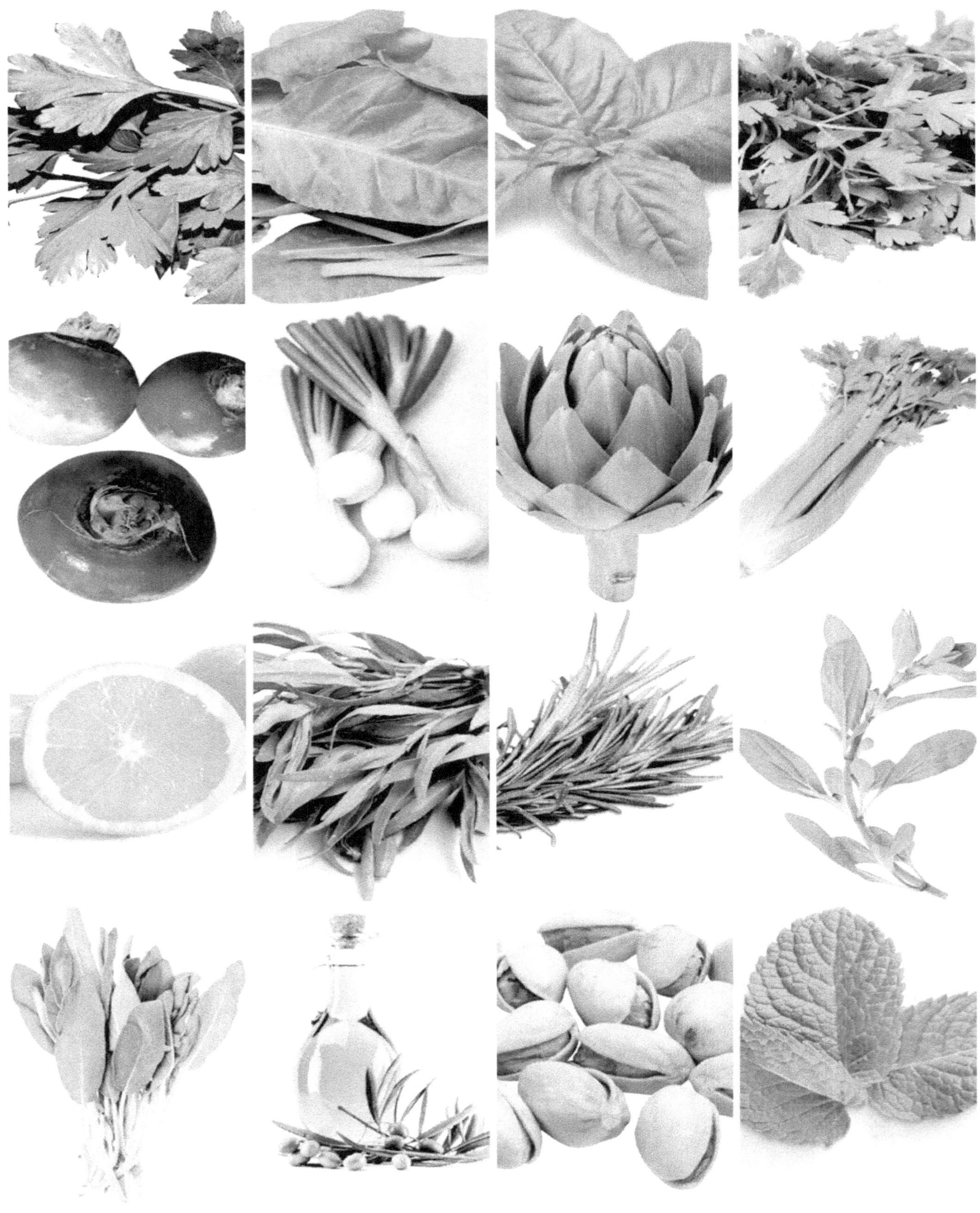

# Hesperetin and Hesperidin

Hesperetin and hesperidin are flavanones found in multiple citrus fruits and herbs, such as peppermint and chrysanthemum. Consuming more hesperetin and hesperidin-rich foods for their antiviral, anti-inflammatory, and immune-modulating effects may also be as important as imbibing herbal remedies. Besides its antioxidant, anti-inflammatory, and immune-modulating effects, you will recall that hesperetin, a flavanone in Pericarpium Citri Reticulatae, is predicted to bind with ACE2 to prevent SARS-CoV-2 entry (Chen & Du, 2020). In addition, hesperidin demonstrates potential as a main protease (Mpro) inhibitor (Khaerunnisa et al., 2020). All of these effects make hesperetin and hesperidin ideal candidates for viral respiration infections.

## Herbs that Contain Hesperetin and Hesperidin

| | |
|---|---|
| • Pericarpium Citri Reticulatae<br><br>• Fructus Aurantii Immaturus | • Herba Menthae<br><br>• Flos Chrysanthemi |

## Foods That Contain Hesperetin and Hesperidin

The following foods contain hesperetin and hesperidin. Interestingly, spring onions and oranges are among the most nutrient-dense foods featured in the Guide to Nutrivore (Ballantyne, 2022).

## Hesperetin and Hesperidin-Rich Foods

| | |
|---|---|
| • Grapes/red wine | • Limes |
| • Spring onions | • Blood oranges |
| • Grapefruits | • Tangerines |
| • Oranges | • Peppermint |
| • Lemons | • Chrysanthemum |

Source: (Ballantyne, 2022, Choy et al., 2019; Phenol Explorer).

Below is a visual guide of hesperetin and hesperidin-rich foods to include in your diet. From top to bottom, this includes red wine, spring onions, grapefruits, lemons, blood oranges, limes, oranges, tangerines, mint, mint tea, chrysanthemum and chrysanthemum tea.

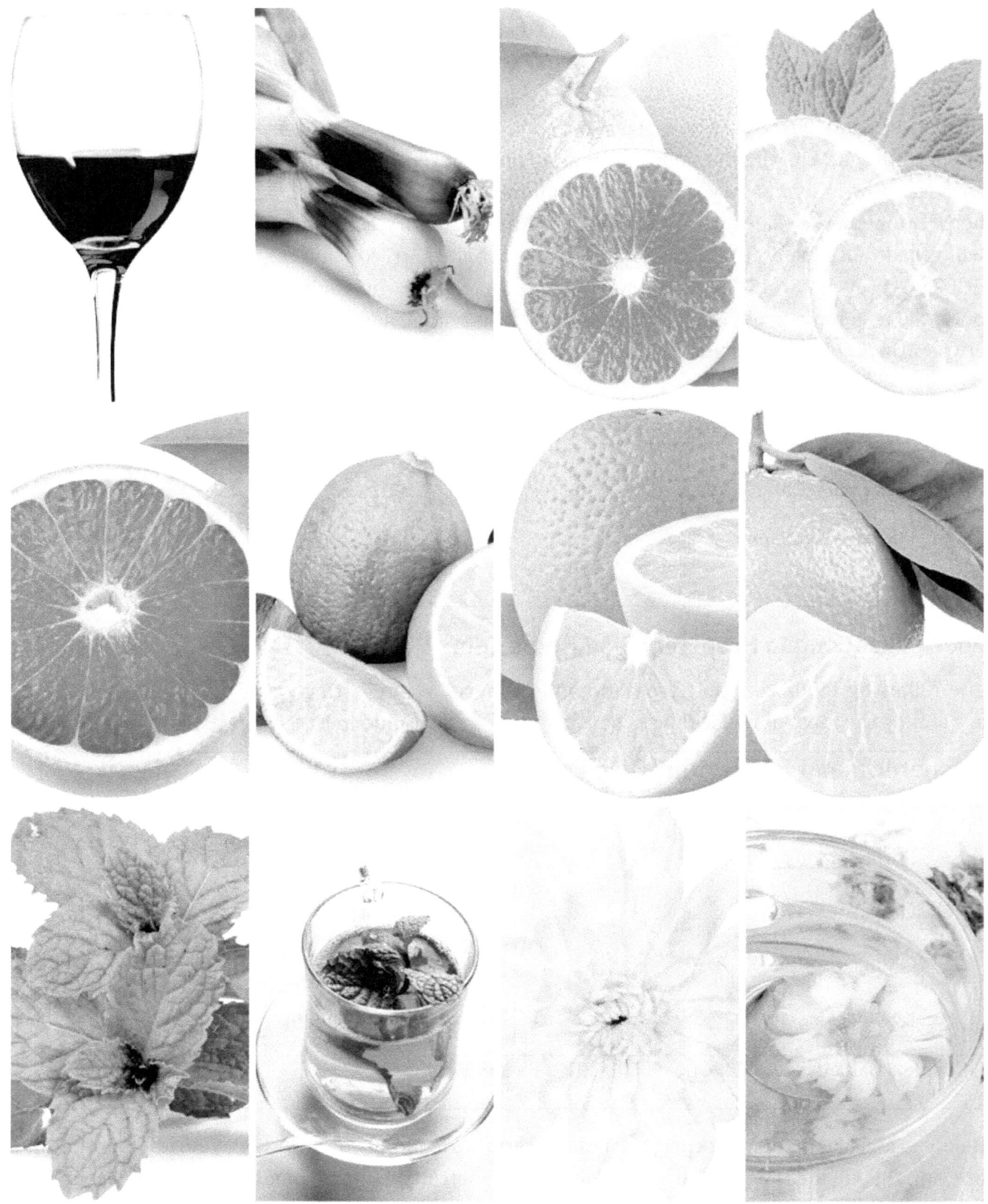

Remember that some plants contain multiple flavonoids, e.g., broccoli, spinach, basil, and mint, all contain luteolin, kaempferol, and quercetin, suggesting their outstanding antiviral, anti-inflammatory, and immune-modulating activity. Given this information, you can appreciate how consuming herbs and foods can help improve host defense against infection. Combining these compounds helps block or inhibit SARS-CoV-2 and decrease NFKB, cytokines, and inflammation, making them outstanding candidates for improving host defenses and helping manage viral respiratory infections.

Now that you know about antiviral, anti-inflammatory, and immune-modulating compounds in herbs and foods, let's continue with a review of the four steps of supportive care that Traditional Chinese Medicine (TCM) practitioners use for viral respiratory infections.

Four Steps of Supportive Care for Viral Respiratory Infections

Traditional Chinese Medicine (TCM) practitioners generally recommend four steps of supportive care when tackling respiratory viruses. The first step is to support the immune system via an improved diet and herbal medicine to improve the host's defense against infection. The second step addresses the early stage of infection. The third step addresses acute symptoms. Finally, the fourth step addresses the recovery phase.

## Step 1- Foods to Support the Immune System

The first step of supportive care is to improve the host's defense against infection. In my practice, self-care tips include adequate hydration, reducing stress, improving sleep, and eating a phytonutrient-rich, anti-inflammatory diet for a balanced immune system.

An anti-inflammatory diet emphasizes phytonutrient-rich fruit and vegetables and animal sources of nutrition that contribute to optimal immune function. For example, selenium can be sourced from cod, shrimp, salmon, tuna, Brazil nuts, and button mushrooms. You can obtain zinc from oysters, crab, lobster, kale, mushrooms, beef, and chicken. Other trace minerals such as iodine, iron, and chromium can be sourced from sea vegetables such as kelp and wakame. Vitamin D can be sourced from cod liver oil, herring, trout, salmon, halibut, mushrooms, and beef liver. Food sources of Vitamin K2 include animal products, fermented foods, and leafy greens such as spinach, kale, and collards (that add K1 for conversion to K2 by your microflora). Vitamin E can be found in avocado and all greens, especially turnip greens.

Meanwhile, methylation factors such as B12 (cobalamin) can be obtained from beef liver, clams, trout, salmon, lamb, halibut, shrimp, and grass-fed beef. Vitamin B6 (pyridoxine) can be sourced from mustard greens, cabbage, cauliflower, kale, broccoli, chard, collard greens, leeks, garlic, tuna, cod, pork, calf's liver, turkey, and salmon. B9 (folate) sources include turnip greens, spinach, romaine lettuce, asparagus, Brussels sprouts, broccoli, sunflower seeds, beans, and fruit.

Magnesium can be found in spinach, chard, beet greens, figs, bananas, almonds, pumpkin seeds, avocados, cocoa, and unsweetened dark chocolate.

## Common Vitamin and Mineral Sources

| | |
|---|---|
| • Selenium | Cod, shrimp, salmon, tuna |
| • Zinc | Oysters, crab, lobster, beef, chicken |
| • Iodine, iron, chromium | Sea Vegetables |
| • Magnesium | Greens, figs, nuts, seeds, cocoa |
| • Vitamin D | Trout, salmon, halibut, beef liver |
| • Vitamin C | Citrus, kiwi, guava, parsley |
| • Vitamin K2 | Animal products, fermented foods |
| • Vitamin B12 | Beef liver, beef, lamb, halibut |
| • Vitamin B6 | Mustard greens, broccoli, tuna |
| • Vitamin B9 | Dark leafy greens, liver, seafood |
| • Vitamin E | All leafy greens |

While micronutrients and macronutrients such as vitamins, minerals, and fats are crucial to building host defenses, it is clear from the research that other key ingredients, especially phytonutrients, are particularly effective for inhibiting viruses through multiple mechanisms of action. For example, we now know that specific flavonoids such as quercetin, kaempferol, luteolin, baicalin, and naringenin, have antiviral, anti-inflammatory, and immune-modulating effects. Foods containing these compounds, such as citrus, mustard greens, and onions, are not only a great source of vitamin C, but also contain multiple flavonoids that have antiviral, anti-inflammatory, and immune-modulating effects. This information can help you prioritize consuming the most potent ingredients to combat viral respiratory infections.

# Supplements

While a phytonutrient-rich diet may be sufficient for most people, some may want to top off their reserves with a few supplements with known antiviral and immune-modulating effects, e.g., vitamin C, D, zinc, and probiotics. We also know that specific compounds such as EPA/DHA from fatty fish, Vitamin D, and probiotics may all help to increase regulatory T-cells, which help balance the immune system. To broadly cover immunocompetency, you might also consider supplemental B vitamins. Interestingly, there is evidence that quercetin, combined with vitamins C and D, can exert a synergistic antiviral effect that may provide an additional therapeutic/preventive option due to overlapping antiviral and immunomodulatory properties (Agrawal et al., 2020). In addition, adequate Vitamin D, magnesium, and B12 may also help prevent the need for oxygen support, intensive care support, or both in COVID-19 patients (Tan et al., 2020). Below is a shopping list to consider when you are at the supermarket.

# Kitchen Meds

**Produce**
- ☐ Spinach
- ☐ Mustard Greens
- ☐ Chard
- ☐ Collards
- ☐ Kale
- ☐ Sorrel
- ☐ Chicory
- ☐ Dandelion
- ☐ Asparagus
- ☐ Broccoli
- ☐ Brussels Sprouts
- ☐ Cauliflower
- ☐ Bok Choy
- ☐ Napa Cabbage
- ☐ Savoy Cabbage
- ☐ Green Cabbage
- ☐ Purple Cabbage
- ☐ Bell peppers
- ☐ Radish
- ☐ Celery
- ☐ Fennel
- ☐ Artichokes
- ☐ Kohlrabi
- ☐ Rutabaga
- ☐ Rhubarb
- ☐ Turnips
- ☐ Green beans
- ☐ Peas, snap, snow
- ☐ Mushrooms, all types
- ☐ Beets
- ☐ Carrots
- ☐ Zucchini
- ☐ Summer squash
- ☐ Sweet Potatoes
- ☐ Pumpkin
- ☐ Squash, butternut
- ☐ Mung beans
- ☐ Tomatoes
- ☐ Tomatillos
- ☐ Leeks
- ☐ Spring onions
- ☐ Green onions
- ☐ Yellow onions
- ☐ Red onions
- ☐ Shallots
- ☐ Garlic
- ☐ Sauerkraut

**Seaweed**
- ☐ Kelp
- ☐ Wakame

**Salad**
- ☐ Radicchio
- ☐ Watercress
- ☐ Arugula
- ☐ Endive
- ☐ Green leaf lettuce
- ☐ Red leaf lettuce
- ☐ Butterhead lettuce
- ☐ Romaine
- ☐ Alfalfa sprouts
- ☐ Radish sprouts

**Herbs**
- ☐ Oregano
- ☐ Chives
- ☐ Cilantro
- ☐ Parsley
- ☐ Sage
- ☐ Thyme
- ☐ Rosemary
- ☐ Basil
- ☐ Dill
- ☐ Tarragon
- ☐ Marjoram
- ☐ Turmeric
- ☐ Ginger
- ☐ Lemongrass

**Spices**
- ☐ Cumin
- ☐ Cloves
- ☐ Caraway
- ☐ Saffron
- ☐ Cinnamon
- ☐ Nutmeg

**Tea**
- ☐ Green Tea
- ☐ Black Tea
- ☐ White Tea
- ☐ Oolong Tea
- ☐ Mint Tea
- ☐ Ginger Tea
- ☐ Chamomile Tea
- ☐ Rhodiola Tea
- ☐ Perilla leaf Tea
- ☐ Chrysanthemum Tea
- ☐ Dandelion Tea
- ☐ Skullcap Tea
- ☐ Licorice Tea
- ☐ Lemon Verbena Tea

**Coffee and Cocoa**
- ☐ Coffee
- ☐ Unsweetened cocoa

**Fruit**
- ☐ Apple/juice
- ☐ Asian Pears
- ☐ LycheeFruit
- ☐ Blackberry
- ☐ Strawberry
- ☐ Cherries
- ☐ Blueberries
- ☐ Elderberry
- ☐ Raspberry/juice
- ☐ Cranberry
- ☐ Golden Kiwi
- ☐ Orange/juice
- ☐ Grapefruit
- ☐ Lemons
- ☐ Limes
- ☐ Figs
- ☐ Grapes
- ☐ Pomegranate/juice
- ☐ Bananas
- ☐ Papaya
- ☐ Mango
- ☐ Starfruit
- ☐ Guava
- ☐ Apricots
- ☐ Peaches
- ☐ Plums
- ☐ Prunes
- ☐ Nectarines
- ☐ Watermelon
- ☐ Capers
- ☐ Avocado/Avocado Oil
- ☐ Olives/Olive Oil

**Nuts and Seeds**
- ☐ Brazil nuts
- ☐ Cashews
- ☐ Chestnuts
- ☐ Hazelnuts
- ☐ Pecans
- ☐ Almonds
- ☐ Pistachio nuts
- ☐ Walnuts
- ☐ Pumpkin seeds
- ☐ Sesame seeds
- ☐ Flax seeds

**Legumes**
- ☐ Lentils
- ☐ Chickpeas
- ☐ Black beans
- ☐ White beans
- ☐ Edamame

**Seafood**
- ☐ Oysters
- ☐ Mackerel
- ☐ Mussels
- ☐ Herring
- ☐ Crab
- ☐ Clams
- ☐ Tuna
- ☐ Squid
- ☐ Salmon
- ☐ Trout
- ☐ Sardines
- ☐ Halibut
- ☐ Shrimp
- ☐ Cod

**Meat**
- ☐ Beef Liver
- ☐ Grass-fed beef
- ☐ Chicken
- ☐ Chicken Liver
- ☐ Pork
- ☐ Lamb
- ☐ Turkey
- ☐ Buffalo

**Supplements**
- ☐ Vitamin C
- ☐ Vitamin D
- ☐ Vitamin B12
- ☐ Magnesium
- ☐ Zinc
- ☐ Probiotics
- ☐ Quercetin
- ☐ EPA/DHA

**Extras:**_______________________________________

___________________________________________________

Now that you know more about foods, herbs, and supplements that can help support the immune system, this next section will review several herbal formulas used in Traditional Chinese Medicine (TCM) for the common cold, influenza, bronchitis, and pneumonia. The same herbal formulas are currently recommended as supportive therapy for COVID-19 patients, mainly due to their high flavonoid and phenolic content. While there are many formulas that herbalists may suggest for each phase of the infection, we will review the most commonly recommended herbal formulas for protecting against and managing viral respiratory infections, with caveats for those with autoimmune conditions. In addition, dietary tips and a few recipes will be given for each stage of viral respiratory infections.

Remember that TCM practitioners respect the ever-changing nature of viral illnesses and know when to modify or change a formula depending on the diagnosis at the time of intake. As such, the most accurate formulas will match the stage of infection and include modifications per patient. That said, if you choose to use Traditional Chinese herbal formulas, it's a good idea to consult with a TCM-trained herbalist to ensure you use the herbs correctly at each stage of infection. In any case, you can focus on consuming more phytonutrient-rich herbs and foods in your diet, as previously discussed.

## Herbs to Support the Immune System

For centuries, people have sought herbal remedies for viral respiratory illnesses, including the common cold, influenza, bronchitis, and pneumonia. Herbal medicine has had such enduring success for these (and other) conditions due to the potent phytonutrients in each remedy, especially terpenoids, flavonoids, and other polyphenolic compounds. Jade Screen Powder (Yu Ping Feng San) is the premier formula Traditional Chinese Medicine (TCM) herbalists recommend for supporting the host immune defense against all viral respiratory infections. Jade Screen Powder may be handy for patients prone to cold and flu viruses, e.g., patients with lymphopenia due to lowered immunity. Jade Screen Powder is also considered an ideal formula for those working indoors. Jade Screen Powder includes Astragalus Membranaceus, Atractylodis Macrocephalae Rhizome, and Ledebouriella Divaricata.

The medicinal herb, Atractylodis Macrocephalae Rhizome, contains the sesquiterpene lactone, atractylon, responsible for its potent antiviral activity (Cheng et al., 2016). Sesquiterpene lactones are a large class of polyphenolic compounds (in food and plants) with various pharmacological activities such as anti-inflammatory, antimicrobial, antioxidant, and antiviral effects (Ozcelik et al., 2009). Ledebouriella Divaricata contains chromones, coumarins, lignans, polyacetylenes, and sterols which possess analgesic, anti-proliferative, antioxidant, and iNOS inhibitory activities (Chin et al., 2011).

Importantly, flavonoids, polysaccharides, and saponins in Astragalus Membranaceus enhance toll-like receptor expression; increase cytokines, T and B lymphocyte production, natural killer cells, and macrophages (Li et al., 2019; Yin et al., 2010; Shi et al., 2014), which can improve host defenses against infection. Even though an enhanced immune response is called for to counter respiratory viruses, Astragalus Membranaceus can increase immune cells that may already get overexpressed in patients with autoimmune diseases. Therefore, those with an autoimmune disease should not use this herb or formulas that contain this herb. However, suppose you work with a TCM trained herbalist. In that case, you can request a custom herbal formula that includes Atractylodis Macrocephalae Rhizome and Ledebouriella Divaricata with herbal substitutes for Astragalus Membranaceus that are high in luteolin, quercetin, and kaempferol. Alternatively, those with autoimmune disease can ask a TCM herbalist about Sang Ju Yin (Mulberry Leaf and Chrysanthemum Decoction) (see below) for protection against respiratory viruses. Below is a list of the three herbal ingredients that comprise Jade Screen Powder.

| **Jade Screen Powder - Ingredients** |
|---|
| • Astragalus Membranaceus*<br><br>• Atractylodis Macrocephalae Rhizome<br><br>• Ledebouriella Divaricata |
| *Avoid the use of this herb in autoimmune conditions |

Below is a summary chart of Jade Screen ingredients, bioactive compounds, and actions. Please note the flavonoid content in this formula plus studies for each herb referenced in the chart below.

| Jade Screen Powder Ingredients, Bioactive Compounds, and Actions | | |
|---|---|---|
| Jade Screen Ingredients | Herb Name | Bioactive Compounds and Actions |
|  | Astragalus Membranaceus* | Astragalus Membranaceus contains kaempferol, luteolin, quercetin, apigenin, rutin, and daidzein. (Bratkov et al., 2016).<br><br>Flavonoids, polysaccharides, and saponins from Astragalus Membranaceus enhance toll-like receptor expression; increase cytokines, T and B lymphocyte production, natural killer cells, and macrophages (Li et al., 2019; Yin et al., 2010; Shi et al., |

| | | 2014). |
|---|---|---|
| | Atractylodis Macrocephalae Rhizome | Atractylodis Macrocephalae Rhizome contains phenolic acids, including caffeic acid, ferulic acid, and protocatechuic acid (Li et al., 2012).<br><br>Atractylodis Macrocephalae Rhizome contains the antiviral sesquiterpene lactone, atractylon (Cheng et al., 2016). |
| | Ledebouriella Divaricata | Ledebouriella Divaricata contains rutin (Kim et al., 2018).<br><br>Ledebouriella Divaricata contains chromones, coumarins, lignans, polyacetylenes, and sterols and possesses analgesic, antiproliferative, antioxidant, and iNOS inhibitory activities (Chin et al., 2011). |
| *Avoid the use of Astragalus Membranaceus in autoimmune conditions | | |

## Step 2 – Herbs for the Early Stage of Infection

### Formula 1- Mulberry Leaf and Chrysanthemum Decoction

Step two addresses headaches, sore throat, cough, fever, myalgia, nausea, and digestive distress. You must begin using herbal medicine for all respiratory viruses as soon as you notice symptoms. In the case of COVID-19, it is also essential to consult with your doctor immediately and run appropriate tests. If your doctor tells you to isolate at home, Mulberry Leaf and Chrysanthemum Decoction (Sang Ju Yin) may be very helpful to have on hand. The Mulberry Leaf and Chrysanthemum Decoction is commonly used by TCM practitioners for viral respiratory infections, including the common cold, influenza, and acute bronchitis (Chen & Hsu, 2020). Mulberry Leaf and Chrysanthemum Decoction can be used for the early phase of viral respiratory infections, e.g., sore throat, headache, runny nose, cough, and/or mild fever. The instruction is to start using these herbs immediately to halt the progression of symptoms. Mulberry Leaf and Chrysanthemum Decoction may also help protect against viral respiratory infections for those who work indoors with others.

Mulberry leaf and chrysanthemum are the chief ingredients in this formula. Mulberry leaf contains quercetin, kaempferol, morin, and rutin, while chrysanthemum contains apigenin, luteolin, quercetin, hesperetin, and hesperidin, all of which are known for their antiviral, immune-modulating, and anti-inflammatory effects. For example, you'll also recall that apigenin, luteolin, quercetin, kaempferol, and hesperidin may help inhibit the main protease (Mpro) of SARS-CoV-2, thereby disrupting viral replication (Khaerunnisa et al., 2020). As you know, these flavonoids also have antioxidant, immune-modulating, and anti-inflammatory effects. In addition, flavonoids in mulberry leaf are predicted to act on the novel coronavirus spike (S2) protein binding site of human ACE2 protein (Niu et al., 2020). Mulberry leaf also contains morin, which has anti-asthmatic, anti-COPD, and anti-allergic activity (Middleton et al., 1992). Given these effects, you can imagine how this formula may help relieve initial symptoms.

The following chart includes all ingredients and bioactive compounds in Mulberry Leaf and Chrysanthemum Decoction (Sang Ju Yin). Please note the flavonoids in this formula and studies for each herb referenced in the chart below. While these herbs are generally considered safe, it's important to consult with an herbalist when using herbal remedies, as individual needs are always considered.

| Mulberry Leaf and Chrysanthemum Ingredients, Bioactive Compounds, and Actions | | |
| --- | --- | --- |
| Ingredients | Herb Name | Bioactive Compounds and Actions |
|  | Folium Mori | Flavonoids: quercetin, kaempferol, rutin, isoquercitrin, and astragalin (Chen et al., 2018; Zhang et al., 2017).<br><br>Morin, another flavonoid, has anti-asthmatic, anti-COPD, and anti-allergic effects (Middleton et al., 1992).<br><br>Flavonoids in Mulberry leaf are predicted to act on the novel coronavirus spike (S2) protein binding site of human ACE2 protein (Niu et al., 2020). |

| | | |
|---|---|---|
| 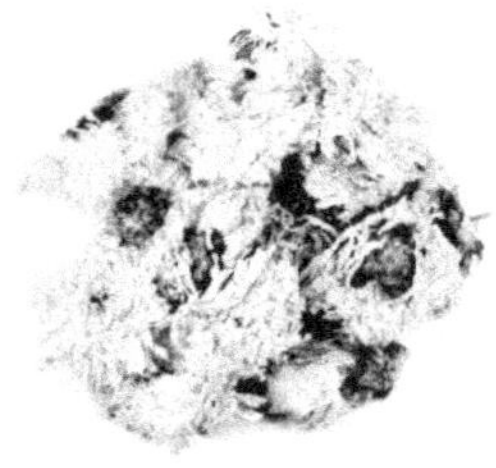 | Flos Chrysanthemi | Flavonoids: Apigenin, luteolin, quercetin, hesperetin, hesperidin (Du et al., 2015).<br><br>Ameliorates acute lung injury via downregulating TLR4/NFKB (Li et al., 2015). |
| 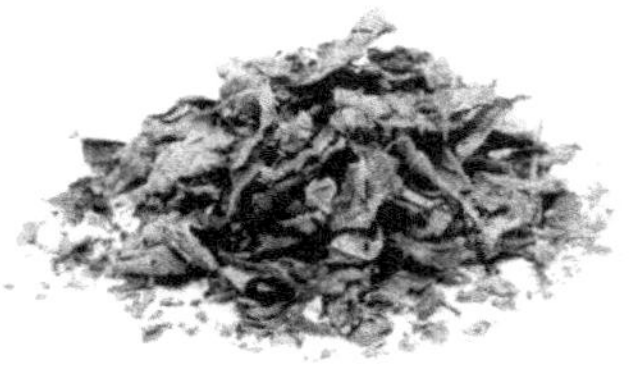 | Herba Menthae | Flavonoids: Quercetin, apigenin, hesperetin, hesperidin (Zhu, 1998).<br><br>Diosmin, another flavonoid, downregulates the expression of T cell receptors, proinflammatory cytokines and NFKB activation against LPS-induced acute lung injury (Imam et al., 2015). |
| 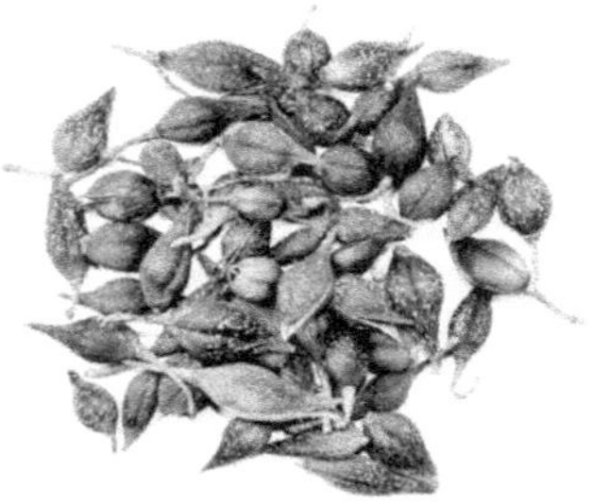 | Fructus Forsythiae | Flavonoids: luteolin, quercetin, kaempferol, rutin, baicalin, and wogonin. Forsythoside A, a polyphenolic compound, has antiviral effects against influenza (Law et al., 2017).<br><br>Lian Qiao (Fructus Forsythiae) could act on the spike (S2) protein binding site of ACE2 to block viral entry of SARS-CoV-2 (Niu et al., 2020; Chan et al., 2020).<br><br>Also contains lignans (forsythin) and triterpenoids (betulinic acid, oleanolic acid, ursolic acid) (Dong et al., 2017). |

51

| | | |
|---|---|---|
| | Radix Platycodi | Platycodin D attenuates acute lung injury by suppressing apoptosis and inflammation in vivo and in vitro (Tao et al., 2015).<br><br>Platycodin D demonstrated high binding affinity to $PL^{pro}$, which is another protease that regulates viral replication in SARS-CoV-2 (Wu et al., 2020). |
| | Armeniacae Amarum | Amygdalin inhibits NFKB and NLRP3 signaling pathways in LPS-induced acute lung injury (Zhang et al., 2017).<br><br>Amygdalin has an antitussive effect (Miyagoshi et al., 1986). |
| | Rhizoma Phragmitis | Contains phenolic acids and lignans (Choi et al., 2014). |

| | Radix Glycyrrhizae | Glycyrrhizin is predicted to bind to the ACE2 receptor to prevent SARS-CoV-2 entry (Chen & Du, 2020).<br><br>Glycyrrhizin inhibits IL-6 in macrophages (Liu et al., 2014).<br><br>Isoliquiritigenin inhibits NFKB activation to suppress the inflammatory response in ARDS (Lago et al., 2014).<br><br>Glycyrrhiza Glabra contains the antiviral triterpenoid, glycyrrhizin, found to inhibit SARS-CoV-1 (Cinatl et al., 2003).<br><br>Licorice root also reduces excessive immune response in those with autoimmune disease and allergies, including allergic asthma (Winston & Maimes, 2007). |
|---|---|---|

Note: Armeniacae Amarum is a tree nut that should be avoided by those with tree nut allergies. If this is the case, a TCM-trained herbalist can recommend an appropriate substitution for you.

## Dietary Support

Dietary support at this stage of the infection includes phytonutrient-rich foods, especially those containing luteolin, apigenin, quercetin, kaempferol, rutin, hesperetin, hesperidin, glycyrrhizin, and others that closely match this formula. For example, consuming broths, leafy greens, onions, berries, citrus, citrus juices, peppermint, chrysanthemum, and licorice teas will improve host defense against infection. That said, it would be prudent to have these items on hand.

# Recipes for Sore Throat, Thirst, and Mild Fever

During this stage, it can be helpful to have plenty of citrus juices high in quercetin, hesperetin, and hesperidin on hand, such as grapefruit and orange juice. In addition, herbal teas with honey will help to soothe a sore throat. Notably, some bioactive compounds in honey, such as chrysin, caffeic acid, galangin, and hesperidin, demonstrate potential antiviral effects, while others (ascorbic acid) enhance antiviral immune responses (Al-Hatamei, 2020). Besides soothing teas, the following flavonoid-rich recipes can help soothe a sore throat and reduce inflammation. In addition, you can diffuse essential oils of lemon, thyme, and peppermint.

## Thai Coconut-Chicken Soup

- 2 lbs. boneless, skinless chicken thighs (diced)
- 1 shallot (minced)
- 1 spring onion (chopped)
- 2 tbsp. garlic (minced)
- 1 tbsp. lime juice
- 1 tbsp. fish sauce
- 2 cups chicken broth
- 2 tsp. fresh grated ginger
- 4-inch piece of fresh lemongrass (chopped)
- 4 green onions (chopped)
- 1 cup of mushrooms (sliced)
- 1 can coconut milk
- ½ cup fresh basil (chopped)
- ½ cup cilantro (chopped)

*Preparation*

1. Add all ingredients to slow cooker and cook for 2 hours on low.
2. Top with green onions, basil, and cilantro.

Servings: 4

### Peppermint, Licorice, and Honey Tea

- 1 peppermint tea bag
- 1 licorice tea bag
- ¼ tsp. honey
- 1 cup boiling water

*Preparation*

1. Add ingredients to a large mug and top with 1 cup of boiling water.

2. Let steep for 5 minutes and enjoy.

Servings: 1

### Peppermint and Chrysanthemum Tea

- 1 dried chrysanthemum flower or teabag
- 1 bag of peppermint tea
- ¼ tsp. honey
- 2 cups boiling water

*Preparation*

1. Add ingredients to a tea pot and top with 2 cups of boiling water.

2. Let steep for 10 minutes, strain chrysanthemum flower and enjoy.

Servings: 1

## Chrysanthemum and Mulberry Leaf Tea

- 1 dried chrysanthemum flower or teabag
- 1 tbsp. dried mulberry leaf or teabag
- ¼ tsp. honey
- 1 cup boiling water

*Preparation*

1. Add ingredients to a teapot and top with 1 cup of boiling water.

2. Let steep for 10 minutes, strain and enjoy.

Servings: 1

## Strawberry, Kiwi, and Mint Sorbet

- Two frozen kiwis

- 10 ounces of frozen strawberries

- ¼ cup of peppermint or spearmint leaves

*Preparation*

1. Place all ingredients in a blender

2.  Blend for 5 minutes

Servings: 2

## Lemon-Orange-Honey Gelatino

- Juice from 1 orange

- 1 tsp. grated lemon zest

- 1 tsp. grated orange zest

- ¼ tsp. honey

- 1 cup boiling water

- 4 tbsp. unflavored gelatin

*Preparation*

1. Mix orange juice, honey, lemon, and orange zest, set aside.

2. Add 1 cup boiling water to 4 tablespoons of gelatin in a bowl.

3. Strain lemon and orange zest from juice and add to gelatin.

4. Pour into a glass dish or molds and refrigerate for 60 minutes.

Servings: 1


Mulberry Leaf and Chrysanthemum Decoction (*Sang Ju Yin*) and dietary support can be helpful for sore throat, thirst, and mild fever. However, if gastrointestinal symptoms are an issue, you can ask your herbalist about Agastache Formula to Rectify the Qi (*Huo Xiang Zheng Qi Wan*) for digestive support.

## Step 2 –Herbs for Headache, Fever, Myalgia, and Digestive Upset

### Formula 2 - Agastache Formula to Rectify the Qi

Agastache Formula to Rectify the Qi (Huo Xiang Zheng Qi Wan) can be used for headaches, fever, myalgia, nausea, vomiting, abdominal pain, and diarrhea. Suppose symptoms such as cough and sore throat co-exist simultaneously. You can combine Agastache Formula to Rectify the Qi (Huo Xiang Zheng Qi Wan) with Mulberry Leaf and Chrysanthemum Decoction (Sang Ju Yin) above. The following chart describes the many bioactive compounds and their actions in Agastache Formula to Rectify the Qi. Please note studies for each herb referenced in the chart below. While all these herbs are generally recognized as safe, it's important to consult with an herbalist when using herbal prescriptions, as individual needs are always considered for each stage of the infection.

Agastache Formula to Rectify the Qi Ingredients, Bioactive Compounds, and Actions

| Ingredients | Herb Name | Bioactive Compounds and Actions |
|---|---|---|
|  | Herba Agastaches Pogostemonis | Contains phenylpropanoids, terpenoids, phenolics, rosmarinic acid, agastachin (Zielińska, & Matkowski, 2014).<br><br>Patchouli alcohol contained Herba Pogostemonis inhibits $M^{pro}$ and, therefore, viral replication of SARS-CoV-2 (Wu et al., 2020).<br><br>Patchouli alcohol in Herba Pogostemonis also acts on the ACE2 receptor to prevent viral entry (Wu et al., 2020).<br><br>Contains pachypodol, a tri-o-methyl ether of quercetin that inhibits several human pathogenic RNA viruses, including rhinovirus, coxsackievirus and poliovirus, acting on viral plus-strand RNA replication (Ishitsuka et al., 1982). |

| | | |
|---|---|---|
| | Radix Glycyrrhizae | Glycyrrhizin is predicted to bind to the ACE2 receptor to prevent SARS-CoV-2 entry (Chen & Du, 2020).<br><br>Glycyrrhizin inhibits IL-6 in macrophages (Liu et al., 2014).<br><br>Isoliquiritigenin inhibits NFKB activation to suppress the inflammatory response in ARDS (Lago et al., 2014).<br><br>Licorice root also reduces excessive immune response in those with autoimmune disease and allergies, including allergic asthma (Winston & Maimes, 2007). |
| | Radix Platycodi | Platycodin D attenuates acute lung injury by suppressing apoptosis and inflammation in vivo and in vitro (Tao et al., 2015).<br><br>Platycodin D demonstrated high binding affinity to PL$^{pro}$ (Wu et al., 2020). |

| | | |
|---|---|---|
| | Cortex Magnoliae Officinalis | Cortex Magnoliae Officinalis contains quercetin, kaempferol magnolol, and honokiol (Rajgopal et al., 2016).<br><br>Aporphine alkaloids were shown to interfere with the viral replicative cycle of poliovirus (Boustie et al., 1998). |
| | Rhizoma Pinelliae Preparata | Baicalein, β-sitosterol, shogaol, and gingerol inhibit NFKB in acute airway viral infections (Eng et al., 2019). |
| | Pericarpium Citri Reticulatae | Pericarpium Citri Reticulatae contains nobiletin which ameliorates inflammation in acute lung injury by suppression of NFKB pathway in vivo and vitro (Li et al., 2018).<br><br>Hesperetin from Pericarpium Citri Reticulatae is predicted to bind with ACE2 (Chen & Du, 2020). |
| | Atractylodis Macrocephalae Rhizome | Atractylodis Macrocephalae Rhizome contains phenolic acids including caffeic acid, ferulic acid, and protocatechuic acid (Li et al., 2012).<br><br>Contains the antiviral sesquiterpene lactone, atractylon (Cheng et al., 2016). |

| | | |
|---|---|---|
| | Sclerotium Poriae Cocos | Poria Cocos Polysaccharide (PCP) has immunomodulatory activity through TLR4, TRAF6, and NFKB signaling both in vitro and in vivo (Tian et al., 2019). |
| | Angelicae Dahuricae Radix | Angelicae Dahuricae Radix has anti-nociceptive and anti-inflammatory effects through inhibition of inducible nitric oxide synthase and NO production (Kang et al., 2008) |
| | Pericarpium Arecae Catechu | Areca catechu plant extracts inhibited syncytium formation, and trafficking of the hemagglutinin-neuraminidase (HN) glycoprotein to the cell-surface in Newcastle disease virus (NDV) (Lee et al., 2014). |
| | Folium Perillae | Folium Perillae contains anthocyanins and anti-inflammatory rosmarinic acid.<br><br>Folium Perillae has anti-allergic, anti-inflammatory, antioxidant, anticancer, antimicrobial, antidepressant, and anti-cough effects (Yu et al., 2017). |
| | Zizyphus Jujubae | Zizyphus Jujubae contains oleanolic acid, betulinic acid, quercetin, apigenin (Eng et al., 2019). |

## Dietary Support

Dietary Support at this stage includes phytonutrient-rich herbs in foods that contain luteolin, apigenin, quercetin, kaempferol, rutin, hesperetin, hesperidin,  and glycyrrhizin. For example, consuming leafy greens, onions, berries, citrus, red dates, ginger, chrysanthemum, peppermint, and licorice teas can help relieve symptoms. That said, it would be prudent to have these items on hand.

## Recipes for Low Appetite, Headache, and Nausea

In addition to herbal remedies, the following flavonoid-rich recipes can help when you have a diminished appetite, upset stomach, or nausea. In addition, you can diffuse essential oils such as ginger and peppermint. You can also experiment with adding one or more herbs from the above formula when cooking. For example, you can add Pericarpium Citri Reticulatae (dried citrus peel), Zizyphus Jujubae (red dates), and ginger (Rhizoma Zingiberis Recens) to your chicken broth. Besides its anti-inflammatory, immune-modulating, and antiviral effects, ginger is a well-known carminative herb that benefits digestion.

## Fresh Ginger, Lemon, and Honey Tea

- Juice from ½ lemon
- ¼ tsp. honey
- 1 tsp. grated ginger
- 1 cup boiling water

*Preparation*

3. Add ingredient to a large mug and top with 1 cup of boiling water.

4. Let steep for 5-10 minutes, strain ginger and liquid into a new mug and enjoy.

Servings: 1

## Peppermint Tea

- 1 peppermint tea bag
- 1 cup boiling water

*Preparation*

1. Add tea bag to a large mug and top with 1 cup of boiling water.
2. Let steep for 5 minutes and enjoy.

Servings: 1

# Medicinal Chicken Bone Broth

- 2 lbs. bony chicken pieces
- 2 peeled and chopped purple or orange carrots
- 1 peeled and chopped daikon radish
- 1 spring onion (chopped)
- 3 thick slices of ginger
- 5 red dates (Zizyphus Jujubae)
- 3 dried citrus peels (Pericarpium Citri Reticulatae)
- 3 quarts of water
- Sea salt to taste
- ¼ bunch fresh thyme leaves

*Preparation*

5. Add veggies, chicken, and herbs to 3 quarts of water in a large pot.
6. Cook for 2 hours on a low boil.
7. When cool, pour through a strainer to enjoy clear broth

Servings: 2

# Carrot-Ginger Soup

- 3 tbsp. olive oil
- 7 large purple or orange carrots, peeled and sliced thin
- 1tsp. ginger (minced)
- 2 cups of vegetable or chicken broth
- 2 cups water
- 1 tbsp. of orange zest
- ½ cup chopped cilantro for garnish
- Sea salt to taste

*Preparation*

1. Sautee carrots in olive oil.
2. Add stock, water, ginger, and orange zest.
3. Bring to a simmer, cover, and cook for 20 minutes.
4. Pour soup in a blender and puree until smooth.
5. Add salt to taste and garnish with cilantro.

Servings: 1—2

## Step 3 - Mitigate Acute Symptoms

Step three addresses acute symptoms, including excessive phlegm, bronchitis, and pneumonia. Once again, it is important to note that herbs are not a substitute for appropriate medical intervention. Always check with your doctor before using herbal medicine.

## Herbs to Alleviate Acute Symptoms

While herbalists use different formulas, Clear the Qi and Transform Phlegm Pill (Qing Qi Hua Tan Wan) may be the most effective for quelling inflammation and resolving phlegm that results from respiratory illness. Clear the Qi and Transform Phlegm Pill has historically been used for cough, excessive phlegm, bronchitis, and pneumonia. The chart below lists all of the herbs in this formula. While these herbs are generally recognized as safe, it's important to consult with a TCM-trained herbalist, as individual needs are always considered.

                                    

| **Clear the Qi and Transform Phlegm Pill - Ingredients** | |
| --- | --- |
| <ul><li>Arisaema</li><li>Rhizoma Pinelliae</li><li>Sclerotium Poriae Cocos</li><li>Scutellariae Baicalensis</li></ul> | <ul><li>Fructus Aurantii Immaturus</li><li>Armeniacae Amarum</li><li>Fructus Trichosanthis</li><li>Pericarpium Citri Reticulatae</li></ul> |

Clear the Qi and Transform Phlegm Pill (Qing Qi Hua Tan Wan) provides potent antiviral, immune-modulating, and anti-inflammatory effects. For example, potent herbal compounds from Rhizoma Pinelliae Preparata, including baicalein, β-sitosterol, shogaol, and gingerol, inhibit NFKB in acute airway viral infections (Eng et al., 2019). Meanwhile, nobiletin, a flavonoid in Pericarpium Citri Reticulatae, ameliorates inflammation in acute lung injury by suppressing the NFKB pathway in vivo and in vitro (Li et al., 2018). In addition, hesperetin, a flavanone in Pericarpium Citri Reticulatae is predicted to bind with ACE2 to prevent SARS-CoV-2 entry (Chen & Du, 2020).

Flavonoids in Scutellaria Baicalensis, including baicalin, chrysin, wogonin, and oroxylin A, demonstrated therapeutic efficacy against acute lung injury caused by influenza A virus (H1N1) (Zhi et al., 2019). Scutellarin, a flavone in Scutellaria Baicalensis, inhibits NFKB and pro-inflammatory cytokines (IL-6, TNF-α, and IL- 1β), suppresses NLRP3 inflammasome activation in macrophages (Liu et al., 2018; Wang et al., 2016; Tan et al., 2016), and protects against lipopolysaccharide (LPS)-induced acute lung injury via inhibition of NFKB activation in mice (Tan et al., 2009). Importantly, scutellarin is also predicted to bind to the ACE2 receptor to prevent SARS-CoV-2 entry (Chen & Du, 2020). These properties make Scutellaria Baicalensis one of the most powerful herbs for treating viral respiratory infections.

Fructus Aurantii Immaturus contains multiple flavonoids, including hesperidin, neohesperidin, hesperetin, rutin, rhoifolin, and naringenin (Bai et al., 2018). You'll recall that hesperidin, neohesperidin, and rutin demonstrate potential as Mpro inhibitors (Khaerunnisa et al., 2020). Meanwhile, Trichosanthis Fructus contains multiple phytonutrients, including terpenoids, phytosterols, flavonoids, and lignans that affect the cardiopulmonary system. Numerous studies have shown that extracts and compounds isolated from Trichosanthis Fructus exhibit pharmacological activities, including protective, anti-hypoxic, anti-platelet aggregation, expectorant, anti-inflammatory, and antioxidant effects (Yu et al., 2019).

Separately, amygdalin in Armeniacae Amarum inhibits NFKB and NLRP3 signaling pathways in LPS-induced acute lung injury (Zhang et al., 2017), which demonstrates its anti-inflammatory activity. In addition, amygdalin has an antitussive effect (Miyagoshi et al., 1986), making it great for excessive coughing. Meanwhile, Arisaema extract has also been shown to decrease pro-inflammatory cytokines IL-1β, IL-6, and TNF-α and suppress LPS-induced iNOS and cyclooxygenase-2 (COX-2) in macrophages (Ahn et al., 2011). Considering the combined effects of these herbs, you can imagine how this formula might help to mitigate acute symptoms of viral respiratory infections.

## Dietary Support

Dietary support at this stage should include phytonutrient-rich herbs and foods that contain baicalein, β-sitosterol, shogaol, gingerol, hesperidin, hesperetin, rutin, rhoifolin, naringenin, and lignans. For example, consuming broths, spring onions, pistachio nuts, walnuts, avocado, ginger, and citrus, along with skullcap, ginger, black, green, and licorice teas may help relieve symptoms. That said, it would be prudent to have these items on hand.

## Recipes for Acute Symptoms

In addition to other healing broths and soups, the following flavonoid-rich recipes can support you during the acute phase of respiratory infections.

## Flavonoid-Rich Veggie Broth

- 1 gallon of water
- 2 sliced purple or orange carrots
- 2 sliced ribs of celery
- 1 cup of chopped daikon radish
- 1 cup of sliced leeks
- 1 cup of green cabbage
- 2 cups of chopped kale
- 4 thick slices of ginger
- 4 thick slices of turmeric

### *Preparation*

1. Place all ingredients in a large pot and place on a low boil for 60 minutes.
2. Cool, strain out veggies, and discard them.
3. Store in fridge. Heat and drink 3-4 cups/day.

Servings: 8 cups

# Multi-Flavonoid Chicken Soup

- 1 spring onion (chopped)
- 2 large orange or purple carrots (chopped)
- 1 cup celery (chopped)
- 1 cup broccoli florets
- 6 garlic cloves (minced)
- 2 tbsp. turmeric (minced)
- 2 lbs. boneless, skinless, chicken thighs
- 6 tbsp. olive oil
- 2 tsp. sea salt
- 6 cups water
- ½ cup of chopped cilantro for garnish

*Preparation*

1. Place olive oil, chicken, spring onion, carrots, cabbage, broccoli, garlic, and turmeric in an Instant Pot.
2. Sauté for 30 minutes, adding water as needed until the chicken is lightly browned.
3. Add 6 cups of water and seal the Instant Pot lid.
4. Select "Soup" and high pressure for 30 minutes.
5. Wait approximately 30 minutes for the pressure to release before opening the lid.
6. Take out the chicken, debone and place the meat back in the Instant Pot. Stir.
7. Serve with chopped cilantro on top.

Servings: 3

## Step 4 - Recovering from Viral Respiratory Infections

Step four addresses digestion, energy, and lung function when recovering from viral respiratory infections. When recovering from respiratory illnesses, especially in acute cases of COVID-19, patients may suffer from pulmonary fibrosis due to lung tissue damage caused by the viral infection and the immune system's response (Spagnolo et al., 2020). In addition, energy will likely be low, and patients may also need support for digestion.

Herbs for the Recovery Phase

If there is scarring of the lung tissue, lung function may also be compromised, leading to symptoms such as wheezing and dyspnea. Patients who still feel weak after recovering from a respiratory infection may benefit from a formula such as Sha Shen Mai Dong Tang (Glehnia and Ophiopogonis Decoction). The chart below lists all of the herbs in Glehnia and Ophiopogonis Decoction. While all these herbs are generally recognized as safe, it's important to consult with an herbalist when using herbs in combination, as individual needs are always considered.

| Glehnia and Ophiopogonis Decoction – Ingredients | |
|---|---|
| • Radix Glehniae | • Dolichoris Lablab |
| • Radix Ophiopogonis | • Radix Trichosanthis |
| • Rhizoma Polygonati Odorati | • Radix Glycyrrhizae |
| • Folium Mori | |

The chief ingredient, Radix Glehniae, has historically been used for cough, blood-streaked sputum, fatigue, dry throat, and thirst. The three main flavonoids in Radix Glehniae include quercetin, isoquercetin, and rutin (Yuan et al., 2002). Other potent compounds in Radix Glehniae include phenylpropanoids, coumarins, lignans, organic acids, terpenoids, polyacetylenes, volatile oils, polysaccharides, and polyols (ibid, 2002). The extract of Radix Glehniae was shown to inhibit the release of nitric oxide (NO), prostaglandin E(2) (PGE(2)), TNF-$\alpha$, IL-1$\beta$, inducible nitric oxide synthase, and cyclooxygenase-2 (Yoon et al., 2010). Other bioactive components in Radix Glehniae, including coumarins and polyacetylenes, have demonstrated antioxidant, blood circulation-promoting, and immunomodulatory properties (Cui et al., 2009).

The main components of Radix Ophiopogonis include homoisoflavonoids and polysaccharides, which exhibit cardiovascular protection, anti-inflammatory, anticancer, antioxidant, immunomodulating, and anti-tussive effects (Chen et al., 2016). Another key ingredient, Folium

Mori (Mulberry leaf), contains multiple functional flavonoids, including quercetin, kaempferol, rutin, isoquercitrin, and astragalin (Chen et al., 2018; Zhang et al., 2017). You'll recall that Folium Mori also contains morin, which has anti-asthmatic, anti-COPD, and anti-allergic effects (Middleton et al., 1992). In addition, flavonoids in Folium Mori are predicted to act on the novel coronavirus spike (S2) protein binding site of human ACE2 protein (Niu et al., 2020).

Similarly, you will recall that glycyrrhizin, the antiviral triterpenoid in Radix Glycyrrhizae (Licorice root), is also predicted to bind to the ACE2 receptor to prevent SARS-CoV-2 entry (Chen & Du, 2020). In addition, glycyrrhizin has been shown to inhibit IL-6 in macrophages (Liu et al., 2014), helping balance the immune system and decrease inflammation. Meanwhile, another flavonoid in licorice root (Radix Glycyrrhizae), isoliquiritigenin, inhibits NFKB activation and the inflammatory response in acute respiratory distress syndrome (ARDS) (Lago et al., 2014). These effects make licorice root an excellent candidate for viral respiratory illness.

Dietary Tips for Recovery

Dietary support at this stage includes phytonutrient-rich herbs and foods, especially those that contain lignans, quercetin, kaempferol, rutin, and glycyrrhizin. For example, beans, leafy greens, broths, onions, berries, citrus, pumpkin seeds, black tea, green tea, and licorice tea can help relieve symptoms. That said, it would be prudent to have these items on hand.

## Recipes for Recovery

In addition to herbal remedies, probiotic drinks, healing broths, soups, and green smoothies are recommended to improve hydration, digestion, energy, and brain function. Staying hydrated is crucial for keeping your bowels moving, especially if you've been self-isolating for days and not drinking enough fluids. Antioxidant and flavonoid-rich green smoothies are also encouraged for improving methylation and clearing brain fog.

## Flavonoid-Infused Bone Broth

- 1 gallon of water
- 2 lbs. beef bones
- 6 cloves of crushed garlic
- 4 thick ½ inch slices of ginger
- 4 thick ½ inch slices of turmeric
- 2 tablespoon apple cider vinegar
- 1 teaspoon sea salt

*Preparation*

1. Place all ingredients in pot and bring the stock to a boil, then reduce the heat to low and allow the stock to cook for 8 -12 hours, adding water as necessary.

2. Allow the stock to cool then strain to discard bones etc. Store your stock in the fridge and use within a few days.

Servings: 6

## Chicken, Kale, Carrot, and Spring Onion Soup

- 1 quart chicken broth

- 1 grilled and sliced chicken breast

- ½ bunch of Dino kale chopped (remove stalks)

- 1 spring onion (chopped)

- 2 tbsp. olive oil

- 1 sliced orange or purple carrot

- ½ bunch cilantro

- Sea salt to taste

*Preparation*

1. Sprinkle sea salt on chicken, spray with olive oil, and grill for 10 minutes on each side.

2. Sauté kale, spring onion, and carrot in olive oil.

3. Stir in the chicken broth; add salt, sliced chicken, and cilantro.

Servings: 2

## Green Smoothie with Kale, Blueberries, and Ginger

- ½ a bunch Dino kale chopped (remove stalks)

- ½-inch ginger

- 1 cup of fresh blueberries

- 5 cups of water

*Preparation*

1.  Add all ingredients into blender.

2.  Blend for 5 minutes.

Servings: 4

## Lemon-Coconut Kefir Water

- 1 quart coconut water

- ½ cup whole lemon

- 3 tbsp. dairy free water kefir grains

*Preparation*

1.  Purchase non-dairy water kefir grains.

2.  Place water kefir grains in coconut water.

3.  Cover and set aside for 24 hours.

4.  Remove the kefir grains.

5.  Puree lemon with coconut kefir water in a blender.

Servings: 4

# Summary of Herbal Remedies

Below is a summary chart of herbal formulas for viral respiratory infections.

| Herbal Remedies to Support the Immune System | |
| --- | --- |
| • Jade Screen Powder | Cold and flu prevention |
| • Mulberry Leaf and Chrysanthemum Decoction | Immune system support |
| • Agastache Formula to Rectify the Qi | Support for digestion |
| • Clear the Qi and Transform Phlegm Pill | Bronchitis, pneumonia support |
| • Glehnia and Ophiopogonis Decoction | Support for recovery |

## Safety of Medicinal Herbs and Phytonutrients

Now that we have explored the benefits of medicinal herbs, we need to consider their safety. Herbs are generally recognized as safe, but there are some precautions. For example, it is important to remember that herbs commonly recommended for viral respiratory infections, such as Echinacea, Astragalus Membranaceus, and Andrographis Paniculata, may increase immune cells that may already get overexpressed in autoimmune disease patients. Therefore, anyone with an autoimmune condition should avoid using these herbs unless recommended by a trained herbalist.

Also, some compounds, such as the flavone baicalin in Huang Qin (Scutellaria Baicalensis), may magnify or oppose the effect of pharmaceuticals and should be carefully evaluated for those on medications (Tian et al., 2013; Fong et al., 2015). Naringenin in grapefruit juice can also interact with several pharmaceutical drugs, including statins, calcium channel blockers, antihistamines, anti-anxiety drugs, immunosuppressive drugs, and antiviral medications for HIV/AIDS. Therefore, you must talk to your physician or pharmacist before increasing the grapefruit or grapefruit juice you regularly consume. Practitioners and patients are also encouraged to check for hidden allergens in the formulas for those with food allergies or sensitivities to ingredients such as the tree nut, Armeniacae Amarum.

# Final Thoughts

Integrative treatments are urgently needed to manage viral respiratory infections in the United States and elsewhere. Considering the infectiousness of SARS-CoV-2 and its various mutations, we should expect COVID-19 to be around forever. As we arrive at this new frontier of viral respiratory infections, diet, herbal medicine, and vaccines will be crucial in managing Covid-19. Since numerous herbs and foods can regulate inflammation and the immune system response while also providing antiviral and organ protective effects, it is time for everyone to take advantage of supportive herbal and dietary therapies for viral respiratory illnesses. Finding the right combination of nutrient-dense, anti-inflammatory, antiviral, and immune-modulating foods, herbs, and vaccines can help you prevent, mitigate, and resolve viral respiratory infections.

Considering the information in this guide, we can all play a more proactive role in preventing or decreasing the severity of symptoms associated with viral respiratory infections that do not require hospitalization. Thank you for taking the time to read Kitchen Meds. Please help me spread the word to anyone who may benefit from this information. If you have any questions, please don't hesitate to contact me via my website, anneangelone.com.

# References


Agrawal, P.K., Agrawal, C., Blunden, G. (2020). Quercetin: Antiviral Significance and Possible COVID-19 Integrative Considerations. Sage Journals. https://doi.org/10.1177/1934578X20976293

Ahn, C. B., & Je, J. Y. (2012). Anti-inflammatory activity of Arisaema Bile in LPS-induced PMA-differentiated THP-1 cells. Immunopharmacology and immunotoxicology, 34(3), 379–384. https://doi.org/10.3109/08923973.2011.608683

Alam, J., Hussain, T., & Pati, S. (2020). Bio-active Compounds (Curcumin, Allicin and Gingerol) of Common Spices used in Indian and South-east Asian Countries Might Protect against COVID-19 Infection: A Short Review. European Journal of Medicinal Plants, 31(20), 65-78. https://doi.org/10.9734/ejmp/2020/v31i2030363

Al-Hatamleh, M., Hatmal, M. M., Sattar, K., Ahmad, S., Mustafa, M. Z., Bittencourt, M. C., & Mohamud, R. (2020). Antiviral and Immunomodulatory Effects of Phytochemicals from Honey against COVID-19: Potential Mechanisms of Action and Future Directions. Molecules (Basel, Switzerland), 25(21), 0. https://doi.org/10.3390/molecules25215017

Avendaño, C., & Menéndez, J.C. in Medicinal Chemistry of Anticancer Drugs (Second Edition), 2015.

Azam, S., Jakaria, M., Kim, I.S., Kim, J., Haque, M., & Choi, D.K. (2019). Regulation of Toll-Like Receptor (TLR) Signaling Pathway by Polyphenols: Focus on TLR4 Signaling. Frontiers in Immunology, 10. 10.3389/fimmu.2019.01000.

Ballantyne, Sarah. (2022). *Guide to Nutrivore*.

Basu, A., Sarkar, A. & Maulik, U. Molecular docking study of potential phytochemicals and their effects on the complex of SARS-CoV2 spike protein and human ACE2. Sci Rep 10, 17699 (2020). https://doi.org/10.1038/s41598-020-74715-4

Bhagwat, S., Haytowitz, D.B., & Holden, J.M. (2011, September). Nutrient Data Laboratory Beltsville Human Nutrition Research Center Agricultural Research Service. U.S. Department of Agriculture.

Boustie, J., Stigliani, J.L., Montanha, J., Amoros, M., Payard, M., & Girre, L. (1998 April) Antipoliovirus structure-activity relationships of some aporphine alkaloids. Journal of Natural Products, 61(4):480-4

Brahmkshatriya, P.P. & Brahmkshatriya, P.S. (2013, May). Terpenes: Chemistry, Biological Role, and Therapeutic Applications. Natural Products. pp. 2665-2691.

Bratkov, V.M., Shkondrov, A.M., Zdraveva, P.K., & Krasteva, I.N. (2016). Flavonoids from the genus Astragalus: Phytochemistry and biological activity. Pharmacognosy Reviews, 10:11-32.

Bruce, D.F., & Grossan, M. (2007). The Sinus Cure. Ballantine Books.

Calderón-Montaño, J.M., Burgos-Morón, E., Pérez-Guerrero, C., & López- Lázaro, M. (2011, April). A review on the dietary flavonoid kaempferol. Mini Reviews in Medical Chemistry, (4):298-344.

Carrasco-Pozo, C., Morales, P., & Gotteland, M. (2013). Polyphenols protect the epithelial barrier function of Caco-2 cells exposed to indomethacin through the modulation of occludin and zonula occludens-1 expression. Journal of agricultural and food chemistry, 61(22), 5291–5297. https://doi.org/10.1021/jf400150p

Cassidy, A., & Minihane, A. M. (2017). The role of metabolism (and the microbiome) in defining the clinical efficacy of dietary flavonoids. The American Journal of Clinical Nutrition, 105(1), 10–22.

https://doi.org/10.3945/ajcn.116.136051

Chan, K.W., Wang, V.T., & Tang, S.C.W. (2020, March). Covid-19: An Update on the Epidemiological, Clinical, Preventive and Therapeutic Evidence and Guidelines of Integrative Chinese–Western Medicine for the Management of 2019 Novel Coronavirus Disease. The American Journal of Chinese Medicine, Vol. 48, No. 3, 1–26.

Chen, Z., Du, X., Yang, Y., Cui, X., Zhang, Z., & Li, Y. (2018). Comparative study of chemical composition and active components against α- glucosidase of various medicinal parts of Morus alba L. Biomedical Chromatography: BMC, 32(11), e4328. https://doi.org/10.1002/bmc.4328

Chen, J., & Hsu, L. (2020). How Covid-19 (2019-nCoV) is Currently Treated in China with TCM. Compiled, Translated and Edited by John K. Chen, Pharm.D., PhD., OMD, LAc. and Lori Hsu, MTOM, MS. TCM Resources for Coping with Covid-19 published on eLotus.org

Chen, H., & Du, Q. (2020). Potential Natural Compounds for Preventing 2019-nCoV Infection. Preprints.org. 2020010358.

Chen, M.H., Chen, X.J., Wang, M., Lin, L.G., Wang, Y.T. (2016). Ophiopogon japonicus—A phytochemical, ethnomedicinal and pharmacological review, Journal of Ethnopharmacology, Volume 181, 2016, Pages 193-213, ISSN 0378-8741,

https://doi.org/10.1016/j.jep.2016.01.037.

Cheng, Y., Mai, J.Y., Hou, T.L., Ping, J., & Chen, J.J. (2016, February). Antiviral activities of atractylon from Atractylodis Rhizoma. Journal of Integrative Medicine, pp: 3704-3710. https://doi.org/10.3892/mmr.2016.5713

Chirumbolo S. (2010). The role of quercetin, flavonols and flavones in modulating inflammatory cell function. Inflammation & allergy drug targets, 9(4), 263–285.

https://doi.org/10.2174/187152810793358741

Choe, J. Y., and Kim, S. K. (2017). Quercetin and ascorbic acid suppress fructose-induced NLRP3 inflammasome activation by blocking intracellular shuttling of TXNIP in human macrophage cell lines. Inflammation 40, 980–994. doi:10.1007/s10753-017-0542-4

Choi, S.E., Yoon, J.H., Park, K.H., Kim, K.Y., Song, Y.J., Jin, H.Y., & Lee, M.W. (2014). Whitening activity of phenolic compounds from rhizome of Phragmites communis. Natural Product Sciences, 20. 269-273.

Chin, Y.W., Jung, Y.H., Chae, H.S., Yoon, K.D., & Kim, J.W. (2011). Anti-inflammatory Constituents from the Roots of Saposhnikovia divaricata.

Bulletin of Korean Chemistry Society, Vol. 32, No. 6 Notes DOI

10.5012/bkcs.2011.32.6.2132

Cinatl, J., Morgenstern, B., Bauer, G., Chandra, P., Rabenau, H., & Doerr, H.W. (2003). Glycyrrhizin, an active component of liquorice roots, and replication of SARS-associated coronavirus. The Lancet, 361:2045-6

Cui H. Y., Xu Y. P. Review of chemical constituents and pharmacological effects of Glehnia littoralis. China Science and Technology Information. 2009;19:203–204.

Dabeek, W.M., and Marra, M.V. (2019, October). Dietary Quercetin and Kaempferol: Bioavailability and Potential Cardiovascular-Related Bioactivity in Humans. Nutrients, (10): 2288. DOI: 10.3390/nu11102288

Das, S., Sarmah, S., Lyndem, S., & Singha Roy, A. (2021). An investigation into the identification of potential inhibitors of SARS-CoV-2 main protease using molecular docking study. Journal of biomolecular structure & dynamics, 39(9), 3347–3357.

https://doi.org/10.1080/07391102.2020.1763201

Ding, S., Jiang, H.M., Fang, J. (2018, April). Regulation of Immune Function by Polyphenols. Journal of Immunology Research. https://doi.org/10.1155/2018/1264074

Dong, Z.L., Lu, X.Y., Tong, X.L., Dong, Y.Q., Tang, L., & Li, M.H. (2017, September).

Forsythiae Fructus: A Review on its Phytochemistry, Quality Control, Pharmacology and Pharmacokinetics. Molecules, 22(9): 1466. DOI: 10.3390/molecules22091466

Du, C.Y., Zheng, K.Y., Bi, C.W., Dong, T.T., Lin, H., & Tsim, K.W. (2015). Yu Ping Feng San, an Ancient Chinese Herbal Decoction, Induces Gene Expression of Anti-viral Proteins and Inhibits Neuraminidase Activity. Phytotherapy Research, 29(5), 656–661.

https://doi.org/10.1002/ptr.5290

Eng, Y.S., Lee, C.H., Lee, W.C., Huang, C.C, & Jung, S.C. (2019). Unraveling the Molecular Mechanism of Traditional Chinese Medicine: Formulas Against Acute Airway Viral Infections as Examples. Molecules, 24, 3505;DOI:10.3390/molecules24193505

Ghezzi, P. (2011, January). Role of glutathione in immunity and inflammation in the lung. International Journal of General Medicine, 4: 105–113. DOI: 10.2147/IJGM.S15618

González, R., Ballester, I., López-Posadas, R., Suárez, M.D., Zarzuelo, A., Martínez-Augustin, O., Sánchez de Medina, F. Effects of Flavonoids and Other Polyphenols on Inflammation. Crit. Rev. Food Sci. Nutr. 2011, 51, 331–362.

Gramza-Michałowska A., Sidor A., Kulczyński B. Berries as a potential anti-influenza factor–A review. J. Funct. Foods. 2017;37:116–137. doi: 10.1016/j.jff.2017.07.050.

Hayashi, Y., Matsushima, M., Nakamura, T., Shibasaki, M., Hashimoto, N.; Imaizumi, K.,...Kawabe, T. (2012). Quercetin protects against pulmonary oxidant stress via heme oxygenase-1 induction in lung epithelial cells. Biochemical and Biophysical Research Communications, 417, 169–174.

Horowitz, R.I., Freeman, P.R., & Bruzzese, J. (2020). Efficacy of glutathione therapy in relieving dyspnea associated with COVID-19 pneumonia: A report of 2 cases. Respiratory medicine case reports, 30, 101063. Advance online publication. https://doi.org/10.1016/j.rmcr.2020.101063

Hu, H.W., Xie, X.M., Zhang, P.Z., & Shu, R.G. (2010). (Study on the flavonoids from Mosla chinensis 'jiangxiangru'). Zhong yao cai = Zhongyaocai Journal of Chinese medicinal materials, 33. 218-9.

Huang F, Li Y, Leung EL, et al. A review of therapeutic agents and Chinese herbal medicines against SARS-COV-2 (COVID-19). Pharmacol Res. 2020;158:104929. doi:10.1016/j.phrs.2020.104929

Huang, Y.F., Bai, C., He, F., Xie, Y., & Zhou, H. (2020). Review on the potential action mechanisms of Chinese medicines in treating Coronavirus Disease 2019 (Covid-19). Pharmacological Research, 104939. Advance online publication. https://doi.org/10.1016/j.phrs.2020.104939

Huang, X.F., Cheng, W.B., Jiang, Y., Liu, Q., Hong, X., Liu, X.H.,...Huang, H.T. (2020, June). A network pharmacology-based strategy for predicting anti-inflammatory targets of ephedra in treating asthma. International Immunopharmacology, Volume 83, 2020, 106423.

Imam F., Al-Harbi, N.O., Al-Harbi, M.M., Ansari, M.A., Zoheir, K.M., Iqbal, M.,...Ahmad, S.F. (2015). Diosmin downregulates the expression of T cell receptors, pro-inflammatory cytokines and NF-κB activation against LPS-induced acute lung injury in mice. *Pharmacology Research*, 102:1–11

Ip, W.K., Chan, K.H., Law, H.K., Tso, G.H., Kong, E.K., Wong, W.H., To, Y.F.,...Lau, Y.L. (2005, May). Mannose-binding lectin in severe acute respiratory syndrome coronavirus infection. *Journal of Infectious Disease*, 15;191(10):1697-704.

Ishitsuka, H., Ohsawa, C., Ohiwa, T., Umeda, I.,  & Suhara, Y. (1982, October) Antipicornavirus flavone Ro 09-0179. Antimicrobial Agents and Chemotherapy, 22(4):611-6.

Kang, O.H., Choi, J.G., Lee, J.H., & Kwon, D.Y. (2010, January). Luteolin Isolated from the Flowers of Lonicera japonica Suppresses Inflammatory Mediator Release by Blocking NF-κB and MAPKs Activation Pathways in HMC-1 Cells. Molecules, 15(1), 385-398;

https://doi.org/10.3390/molecules15010385

Kang, O.H., Chae, H.S., Oh, Y.C., Choi, J.G., Lee, Y.S., Jang, H.J.,...Kwon, D.Y. (2008). Anti-nociceptive and anti-inflammatory effects of Angelicae dahuricae radix through inhibition of the expression of inducible nitric oxide synthase and NO production. American Journal of Chinese Medicine, 36(5):913-28.

Khaerunnisa, S., Kurniawan, H., Awaluddin, R., Suharta, S., & Soetjipto, S. (2020, March). Potential Inhibitor of Covid-19 Main Protease (Mpro) from Several Medicinal Plant Compounds in Molecular Docking Study. Preprints.org. [Epub ahead of print]

Kim, D., Kang, Y.M., Jin, W.Y., Sung, Y., Choi, G., & Kim, H.K. (2014). Antioxidant activities and polyphenol content of Morus alba leaf extracts collected from varying regions. Biomedical Reports, 2, 675-680. https://doi.org/10.3892/br.2014.294

Kun, Wu. (1584). Yi Fang Kao (Investigations of Medical Formulas).

Kuo, M.Y., Liao, M.F., Chen, F.L., Li, Y.C., Yang, M.L., Lin, R.H., & Kuan, Y.H. (2011). Luteolin attenuates the pulmonary inflammatory response involves abilities of antioxidation and inhibition of MAPK and NFkappaB pathways in mice with endotoxin-induced acute lung injury. Food Chemistry and Toxicology, 49, 2660–2666.

Lago, J.H.G., Toledo-Arruda, A.C., Mernak, M., Barrosa, K.H., Martins, M.A., Tibério L.F.L.C., & Prado C.M. (2014). Structure-Activity Association of Flavonoids in Lung Diseases. Brazil Molecules, 19(3), 3570- 3595; https://doi.org/10.3390/molecules19033570

Law, H.Y., Yang, L.H., Lau, S.Y., & Chan, G.C. (2017). Antiviral effect of forsythoside A from Forsythia suspensa (Thunb.) Vahl fruit against influenza A virus through reduction of viral M1 protein. Journal of Ethnopharmacology, 209: 236-247.

Lee, D.S., Boo, K.H., & Kim, Y.C. (2014, April). The Effects of Areca catechu L. Extract. Korean Journal of Food Science and Technology, 46(2):245-248. DOI: 10.9721/KJFST.2014.46.2.245

Li, X., Lin, J., Han, W., Mai, W., Wang, L., Li, Q.,…Chen, D. (2012). Antioxidant ability and mechanism of rhizoma Atractylodes macrocephala. Molecules (Basel, Switzerland), 17(11), 13457–13472.

https://doi.org/10.3390/molecules171113457

Li, Z.X., Zhao, G.D., & Xiong, W. (2019). Immunomodulatory effects of a new whole ingredients extract from Astragalus: a combined evaluation on chemistry and pharmacology. Chinese Medicine, 14, 12. https://doi.org/10.1186/s13020-019-0234-0

Li, C.W., Chen, Z.W., Wu, X.L., Ning, Z.X., Su, Z.Q., Li, Y.C., & Lai, X.P. (2015, March). A Standardized Traditional Chinese Medicine Preparation Named Yejuhua Capsule Ameliorates Lipopolysaccharide-Induced Acute Lung Injury in Mice via Downregulating Toll-Like Receptor 4/Nuclear Factor- κ B. Evidence-Based Complementary and Alternative Medicine, 264612. 10.1155/2015/264612.

Li, W., Zhao, R., Wang, X., Liu, F., Zhao, J., Yao, Q.,…Niu, X. (2018). Nobiletin-ameliorated lipopolysaccharide-induced inflammation in acute lung injury by suppression of NF-kappaB pathway in vivo and vitro. Inflammation, 41 (3), pp. 996-1007.

Li, S., Cheng, C. S., Zhang, C., Tang, G. Y., Tan, H. Y., Chen, H. Y., Wang, N., Lai, A. Y., & Feng, Y. (2021). Edible and Herbal Plants for the Prevention and Management of COVID-19. Frontiers in pharmacology, 12, 656103. https://doi.org/10.3389/fphar.2021.656103

Liang, Y. C., Huang, Y. T., Tsai, S. H., Lin-Shiau, S. Y., Chen, C. F., & Lin, J. K. (1999). Suppression of inducible cyclooxygenase and inducible nitric oxide synthase by apigenin and related flavonoids in mouse macrophages. Carcinogenesis, 20(10), 1945–1952.

https://doi.org/10.1093/carcin/20.10.1945

Liu, H., Ye, F., Sun, Q., Liang, H., Li, C., Li, S., Lu, R., Huang, B., Tan, W., & Lai, L. (2021). Scutellaria baicalensis extract and baicalein inhibit replication of SARS-CoV-2 and its 3C-like protease in vitro. Journal of enzyme inhibition and medicinal chemistry, 36(1), 497–503.

https://doi.org/10.1080/14756366.2021.1873977

Liu, Z., Zhong, J. Y., Gao, E. N., & Yang, H. (2014). Effects of glycyrrhizin acid and licorice flavonoids on LPS-induced cytokines expression in macrophage. Zhongguo Zhong yao za zhi = Zhongguo zhongyao zazhi = China journal of Chinese Materia Medica, 39(19), 3841–3845.

Mashhadi, N. S., Ghiasvand, R., Askari, G., Hariri, M., Darvishi, L., & Mofid, M. R. (2013). Anti-oxidative and anti-inflammatory effects of ginger in health and physical activity: review of current evidence. International journal of preventive medicine, 4(Suppl 1), S36–S42.

Maurya VK, Kumar S, Prasad AK, Bhatt ML, Saxena SK. Structure-based drug designing for potential antiviral activity of selected natural products from Ayurveda against SARS-CoV-2 spike glycoprotein and its cellular receptor. Virus Disease. 2020;31(2):179–193

McKee, D. L., Sternberg, A., Stange, U., Laufer, S., and Naujokat, C. (2020). Candidate Drugs against SARS-CoV-2 and COVID-19. Pharmacol. Res. 157, 104859. doi:10.1016/j.phrs.2020.104859

Middleton, E., & Kandaswami, C. (1992). Effects of flavonoids on immune and inflammatory cell functions. Biochemical Pharmacology, 43, 1167– 1179.

Miean, K.H. & Mohamed, S. (2001). Flavonoid (Myricetin, Quercetin, Kaempferol, Luteolin, and Apigenin) Content of Edible Tropical Plants. Journal of Agricultural and Food Chemistry, 49 (6), 3106-3112, DOI: 10.1021/jf000892m

Miyagoshi, M., Amagaya, S., & Ogihara, Y. (1986) Antitussive effects of L- ephedrine, amygdalin, and makyokansekito (Chinese traditional medicine) using a cough model induced by sulfur dioxide gas in mice. Planta Medica, 4, 275–278.

Niu, M., Wang, R.L., Wang, Z.X., Zhang, P., Bai, Z.F., Jing, J.,... Xiao, X.H. (2020, March). Rapid establishment of traditional Chinese medicine prevention and treatment of 2019-nCoV based on clinical experience and molecular docking. Zhongguo Zhong Yao Za Zhi, 45(6):1213-1218. DOI: 10.19540/j.cnki.cjcmm.20200206.501.

Ozçelik, B., Gürbüz, I., Karaoglu, T., & Yeşilada, E. (2009). Antiviral and antimicrobial activities of three sesquiterpene lactones from Centaurea solstitialis L. ssp. solstitialis. Microbiological Research, 164:545–552. 2009.

Patel, V.J., Biswas, R., Mehta, H.J., Joo, M., & Sadikot, R.T. (2018). Alternative and natural therapies for acute lung injury and acute respiratory distress syndrome. BioMed Research International, Article 2476824

Peng, M., Watanabe, S., Chan, K.W.K., He, Q., Zhao, Y., Zhang, Z.,...Li G (2017, July). Luteolin restricts dengue virus replication through inhibition of the proprotein convertase furin. Antiviral Research, 143:176-185. DOI: 10.1016/j..2017.03.026.

Rajgopal, A., Missler, S. R., & Scholten, J. D. (2016). Magnolia officinalis (Hou Po) bark extract stimulates the Nrf2-pathway in hepatocytes and protects against oxidative stress. Journal of Ethnopharmacology, 193, 657–662. https://doi.org/10.1016/j.jep.2016.10.016

Ren, X., Shao, X.-X., Li, X.-X., Jia, X.-H., Song, T., Zhou, W.-Y., et al. (2020). Aug 10)Identifying Potential Treatments of COVID-19 from Traditional Chinese Medicine (TCM) by Using a Data-Driven Approach. J. Ethnopharmacol. 258, 112932. doi:10.1016/j.jep.2020.112932

Sahoo, M., Jena, L., Rath, S.N., & Kumar, S. (2016). Identification of Suitable Natural Inhibitor against Influenza A (H1N1) Neuraminidase Protein by Molecular Docking. Genomics and Informatics, 14, 96–103.

Santangelo, C., Varì, R., Scazzocchio, B., Di Benedetto, R., Filesi, C., & Masella, R. (2007). Polyphenols, intracellular signaling and inflammation. Annali Dell'Istituto Superiore Di Sanita, 43(4), 394–405.

Schwarz, S., Sauter, D., Wang, K., Zhang, R.H., Sun, B., Karioti, A.,... Schwarz, W. (2014, February). Kaempferol Derivatives as antiviral drugs against the 3a Channel Protein of Coronavirus. Planta Medica, 80(02-03): 177–182. DOI: 10.1055/s-0033-1360277

Shi, L.H., Yin, F.L., Xin, X.G., Mao, S.M., Hu, P.P, Zhao, C.Z., & Sun, X.N. (2014). Astragalus Polysaccharide Protects Astrocytes from Being Infected by HSV-1 through TLR3/NF-κB Signaling Pathway. Evidence Based Complementary and Alternative Medicine, 285356.

https://doi.org/10.1002/bmc.3055

Shi, H., He, J., Li, X., Han, J., Wu, R., Wang, D., et al. (2018). Isorhamnetin, the Active Constituent of a Chinese Herb Hippophae Rhamnoides L, Is a Potent Suppressor of Dendritic-Cell Maturation and Trafficking. Int. Immunopharmacol. 55, 216–222. doi:10.1016/j.intimp.2017.12.014

Singdevsachan S. K., Auroshree P., Mishra J., Baliyarsingh B., Tayung K., Thatoi H. (2016). Mushroom polysaccharides as potential prebiotics with their antitumor and immunomodulating properties: a review. Bioactive Carbohydr. Diet. Fibr. 7, 1–14. 10.1016/j.bcdf.2015.11.001

Song J.-M., Lee K.-H., Seong B.-L. Antiviral effect of catechins in green tea on influenza virus. Antivir. Res. 2005;68:66–74. doi: 10.1016/j.antiviral.2005.06.010.

Spagnolo, P., Balestro E., Aliberti, S., Cocconcelli, E., Biondini, D., Casaet, G.,...Maher, T. (2020, May). Pulmonary fibrosis secondary to COVID- 19: a call to arms? The Lancet, Respiratory Medicine. DOI:https://doi.org/10.1016/S2213-2600(20)30222-8

Suzuki, Y.J., Aggarwal, B.B., & Packer, L. (1992) Alpha-lipoic acid is a potent inhibitor of NF-kappa B activation in human T cells. Biochemistry and Biophysics Research Communications, 189(3):1709–1715. DOI: 10.1016/0006-291x(92)90275-p.

Tallei, T.E, Tumilaar, S.G., Niode, N.J., Fatimawali, Kepel, B.J., Idroes, R. Effendi, Y., Sakib, S.A., Bin Emran, T. "Potential of Plant Bioactive Compounds as SARS-CoV-2 Main Protease ($M^{pro}$) and Spike (S) Glycoprotein Inhibitors: A Molecular Docking Study", Scientifica, vol. 2020, Article ID 6307457, 18 pages, 2020. https://doi.org/10.1155/2020/6307457

Tan, C. W., Ho, L. P., Kalimuddin, S., Cherng, B., Teh, Y. E., Thien, S. Y., Wong, H. M., Tern, P., Chandran, M., Chay, J., Nagarajan, C., Sultana, R., Low, J., & Ng, H. J. (2020). Cohort study to evaluate the effect of vitamin D, magnesium, and vitamin B12 in combination on progression to severe outcomes in older patients with coronavirus (COVID-19). Nutrition (Burbank, Los Angeles County, Calif.), 79-80, 111017. https://doi.org/10.1016/j.nut.2020.111017

Tang, W. *(1798). Wen Bing Tiao Bian* (Systematic Differentiation of Warm Disease). n.p.

Tao, W., Su, Q., Wang, H., Guo, S., Chen, Y., Duan, J., & Wang, S. (2015). Platycodin D attenuates acute lung injury by suppressing apoptosis and inflammation in vivo and in vitro. International Immunopharmacology, 27 (1) pp. 138-147.

Tian, C., Shao, Y., Jin, Z., Liang, Y., Li, C., Qu, C., Sun, S., Cui, C., & Liu, M. (2022). The protective effect of rutin against lipopolysaccharide induced acute lung injury in mice based on the pharmacokinetic and pharmacodynamic combination model. Journal of pharmaceutical and biomedical analysis, 209, 114480.

https://doi.org/10.1016/j.jpba.2021.114480

Tian, H., Liu, Z.J., Pu, Y.W., & Bao, Y.X. (2019, April). Immunomodulatory effects exerted by Poria Cocos polysaccharides via TLR4/TRAF6/NF-κB signaling in vitro and in vivo. Biomedicine and Pharmacotherapy, 112:108709. DOI:10.1016/j.biopha.2019.108709.

Verbeek R, Plomp AC, van Tol EA, van Noort JM. The flavones luteolin and apigenin inhibit in vitro antigen-specific proliferation and interferon-gamma production by murine and human autoimmune T cells. Biochem Pharmacol. (2004) 68:621–9. doi: 10.1016/j.bcp.2004.05.012

Winston, D., & Maimes, S. (2007). Adaptogens: Herbs for strength, stamina, and stress relief. Rochester, VT: Healing Arts Press.

Wu, C.R., Yang, L., Yang, Y.Y., Zhang, P., Zhong, W., Wang, Y.L.,...Li, H. (2020, February) Analysis of therapeutic targets for SARS-CoV-2 and discovery of potential drugs by computational method. Acta Pharmaceutica Sinica B. https://doi.org/10.1016/j.apsb.2020.02.008

Xu, Z., Yang, L., Zhang, X., Zhang, Q., Yang, Z., Liu, Y., Wei, S., & Liu, W. (2020). Discovery of Potential Flavonoid Inhibitors Against COVID-19 3CL Proteinase Based on Virtual Screening Strategy. Frontiers in molecular biosciences, 7, 556481. https://doi.org/10.3389/fmolb.2020.556481

Yang, Q.S., He, L.P., Zhou, X.L., Zhao, Y., Shen, J., Xu, P., & Ni, S.Z. (2015) Kaempferol pretreatment modulates systemic inflammation and oxidative stress following hemorrhagic shock in mice. Chinese Medicine, 10:6.

Yeh, C. H., Yang, J. J., Yang, M. L., Li, Y. C., & Kuan, Y. H. (2014). Rutin decreases lipopolysaccharide-induced acute lung injury via inhibition of oxidative stress and the MAPK-NF-κB pathway. Free radical biology & medicine, 69, 249–257. https://doi.org/10.1016/j.freeradbiomed.2014.01.028

Yuan Z., Tezuka Y., Fan W., Kadota S., Li X. Constituents of the underground parts of Glehnia littoralis. Chemical and Pharmaceutical Bulletin. 2002;50(1):73–77. doi: 10.1248/cpb.50.73.

Yi, L., Li, Z.G., Yuan, K.H., Qu, X.X., Chen, J., Wang, G.W.,... Xia, X.J. (2004). Small molecules blocking the entry of severe acute respiratory syndrome coronavirus into host cells. Journal of Virology, 78:11334-9.

Yin, X.L., Chen, L., Liu, Y., Yang, J.L., Ma, C.Q, Yao, Z.Y.,...Li, M.Y. (2010). Enhancement of the innate immune response of bladder epithelial cells by Astragalus polysaccharides through upregulation of TLR4 expression. Biochemical and Biophysical Research Communications, 397(2):232–8.

Yoon, J. H., & Baek, S. J. (2005). Molecular targets of dietary polyphenols with anti-inflammatory properties. Yonsei Medical Journal, 46(5), 585– 596. https://doi.org/10.3349/ymj.2005.46.5.585

Yu, H., Qiu, J.F., Ma, L.J., Hu, Y.J., Li, P., & Wan, J.B. (2017, October) Phytochemical and phytopharmacological review of Perilla frutescens L. (Labiatae), a traditional edible-medicinal herb in China Food and Chemical Toxicology, Volume 108, Part B, pp. 375-391.

Yu, X., Tang, L., Wu, H., Zhang, X., Luo, H., Guo, R., Xu, M., Yang, H., Fan, J., Wang, Z., & Su, R. (2018). Trichosanthis Fructus: botany, traditional uses, phytochemistry and pharmacology. Journal of ethnopharmacology, 224, 177–194. https://doi.org/10.1016/j.jep.2018.05.034

Zakaryan, H., Arabyan, E., Oo, A., & Zandi, K. (2017, September). Flavonoids: promising natural compounds against viral infections. Archives of Virology, 162(9):2539-2551.

Zhang, D., Li, S., Wang, N., Tan, H. Y., Zhang, Z., & Feng, Y. (2020). The Crosstalk Between Gut Microbiota and Lungs in Common Lung Diseases. Frontiers in Microbiology, 11, 301. https://doi.org/10.3389/fmicb.2020.00301

Zhang, L.W., Ji, T., Su, S. L., Shang, E. X., Guo, S., Guo, J. M.,...Duan, J. A. (2017). Pharmacokinetics of Mori Folium Flavones and Alkaloids in Normal and Diabetic Rats. Zhongguo Zhong yao za zhi = Zhongguo zhongyao zazhi = China journal of Chinese materia medica, 42(21), 4218– 4225. https://doi.org/10.19540/j.cnki.cjcmm.20170901.008

Zhu, Y.P. (1998). Chinese Materia Medica: Chemistry, Pharmacology and Applications. CRC Press.

Zielińska, S., & Matkowski, A. (2014). Phytochemistry and bioactivity of aromatic and medicinal plants from the genus Agastache (Lamiaceae). Phytochemistry Review, 13(2): 391–416. Apr 3. DOI: 10.1007/s11101-014-9349-1

Zuo, G.Y., Li, Z.Q., Chen, L.R., & Xu, X.J. (2007). Activity of compounds from Chinese herbal medicine Rhodiola kirilowii (Regel), Maxim against hcV nS3 serine protease. Antiviral Research, 76:86-92.

## More by Anne Angelone

Safe Supplements for Autoimmune Disease (free)

Gut Clear (free)

The Autoimmune Brain Balance Project

The Paleo Breakthrough Kit

The Secret Sound Healing Project

The Emo-Sensory Project

**Autoimmune Brain and Body Therapy**

Gifted Intelligence

If The Buddha Had an Autoimmune Disease

The Autoimmune Personality

Type G Personality

Beyond Cannabis

The Ego Cure

Functional Scalp Acupuncture

Functional Herbal Medicine and Phytonutrition

Impervious Herbs

**The B27 Diet**